T0227164

Plastic and Reconstructive Surgery

Guest Editor

DEBORAH S. HICKMAN MATHIS, RN, MS, CNOR, RNFA

PERIOPERATIVE NURSING CLINICS

www.periopnursing.theclinics.com

Consulting Editor

NANCY GIRARD, PhD, RN, FAAN

June 2011 • Volume 6 • Number 2

SAUNDERS an imprint of ELSEVIER, Inc.

W.B. SAUNDERS COMPANY

A Division of Elsevier Inc.

1600 John F. Kennedy Boulevard • Suite 1800 • Philadelphia, Pennsylvania 19103-2899

http://www.periopnursing.theclinics.com

PERIOPERATIVE NURSING CLINICS Volume 6, Number 2

June 2011 ISSN 1556-7931, ISBN-13: 978-1-4557-7988-8

Editor: Katie Hartner
Developmental Editor: Donald Mumford

Perioperative Nursing Clinics (ISSN 1556-7931) is published quarterly by Elsevier, 360 Park Avenue South, New York, NY 10010. Months of issue are March, June, September and December. Business and Editorial Offices: 1600 John F. Kennedy Blvd., Suite 1800, Philadelphia, PA 19103-2899. Customer Service Office: 11830 Westline Industrial Drive, St. Louis, MO 63146. Periodicals postage paid at New York, NY and at additional mailing offices. Subscription prices are $124.00 per year (domestic individuals), $213.00 per year (domestic institutions), $61.00.00 per year (domestic students/residents), $161.00 per year (international individuals), $245.00 per year (international institutions), and $65.00 per year (International students/residents). Foreign air speed delivery is included in all *Clinics* subscription prices. All prices are subject to change without notice. **POSTMASTER:** Send change of address to *Perioperative Nursing Clinics*, Customer Service (orders, claims, online, change of address): Elsevier Periodicals Customer Service, 11830 Westline Industrial Drive, St. Louis, MO 63146. Tel: 1-800-654-2452 (U.S. and Canada). Fax: 314-523-5170. E-mail: journals customerservice-usa@elsevier.com (for print support); journalsonlinesupport-usa@elsevier.com (for online support).

Reprints. For copies of 100 or more, of articles in this publication, please contact the Commercial Rights Department, Elsevier Inc., 360 Park Avenue South, New York, NY 10010-1710; Phone: (+1) 212-633-3813; Fax: (+1) 212-462-1935; E-mail: reprints@elsevier.com.

Printed and bound by CPI Group (UK) Ltd, Croydon, CR0 4YY
Transferred to Digital Print 2011

Contributors

CONSULTING EDITOR

NANCY GIRARD, PhD, RN, FAAN
Nurse Collaborations, Boerne, Texas; Clinical Associate Professor, Acute Nursing Care
Department, University of Texas Health Science Center, San Antonio, Texas

GUEST EDITOR

DEBORAH S. HICKMAN MATHIS, RN, MS, CNOR, RNFA
Renue Plastic Surgery, Renue Surgery Center, Brunswick, Georgia

AUTHORS

ANDREA FASSIOTTO, RN
Outpatient Surgery Staff Nurse, Murray Calloway County Hospital, Murray, Kentucky

ALBERTO GOLDMAN, MD
Clinica Goldman of Plastic Surgery, Porto Alegre, Brazil

ROBERT H. GOTKIN, MD, FACS
Cosmetique Dermatology, Laser and Plastic Surgery, LLP, New York, New York

MARK S. GRANICK, MD
Professor and Chief, Division of Plastic Surgery, Department of Surgery, New Jersey
Medical School—UMDNJ, Newark, New Jersey

STEFAN O.P. HOFER, MD, PhD, FRCS(C)
Wharton Chair in Reconstructive Plastic Surgery; Associate Professor, University of
Toronto; Chief, Division of Plastic Surgery, Departments of Surgery and Surgical
Oncology, University Health Network, Toronto, Ontario, Canada

ERIK A. HOY, BS
Medical Student, New Jersey Medical School—UMDNJ, Newark, New Jersey

DEBORAH S. HICKMAN MATHIS, RN, MS, CNOR, RNFA
Renue Plastic Surgery, Renue Surgery Center, Brunswick, Georgia

MARC A.M. MUREAU, MD, PhD
Assistant Professor and Head, Oncological Reconstructive Surgery, Department of Plastic
and Reconstructive Surgery, Erasmus University Medical Center, Rotterdam,
The Netherlands

THERESA (TESS) M. PAPE, PhD, RN, CNOR
Associate Professor, Texas Woman's University College of Nursing, Denton, Texas

JUDITH SELTZER, MS, BSN, RN, CNOR
Molnlycke Health Care, Fallston, Maryland

PAIGE TELLER, MD
Department of Surgical Oncology, Emory University, Atlanta, Georgia

MARY TSCHOI, MD
Resident, Division of Plastic Surgery, Department of Surgery, New Jersey Medical School—UMDNJ, Newark, New Jersey

THERESE K. WHITE, MD, FACS
Plastic and Hand Surgical Associates, South Portland, Maine

Contents

The Institute of Medicine provided the impetus for error awareness in health care organizations with its landmark study of 1999. Since then, societal pressures have increased the momentum for improvements in patient safety. Perioperative errors are often the result of system problems instead of people problems. These can lead to patient injury, increased hospital costs, and blaming others. The error concerns in the perioperative setting include: distractions, interruptions, lack of focus, poor communication, and failure to follow standard procedures. All of this can make for an unsafe environment for patients. Understanding the role of these issues in terms of human factor approaches may provide the impetus for interventions that promote error prevention. Human factors and science and safety strategies borrowed from aviation are described in an effort to shed light on ways to prevent errors within the perioperative setting.

There are multiple ways in which skin preparation can be accomplished. In addition, with the number of skin preparation agents approved for use, nurses sometimes find themselves asking which skin preparation agent will provide the best efficacy for skin disinfection. Adopting a standardized method for selecting and applying the surgical skin preparation may be the best way the surgical team can determine that all patients are receiving the same standard of care, thus promoting best outcomes in their fight against surgical-site infections.

One of the most important tasks of the perioperative nurse is to obtain a thorough history and physical assessment before surgery. The nurse should be able to assess the patient, obtain a history of the patient, and observe for any potential problems.

In the United States, as in many other countries, liposuction is the most commonly performed cosmetic surgical procedure. Advances in technology have enabled surgeons to improve the safety and efficacy of the procedure. One such technological advance is laser-assisted liposuction. This minimally invasive technique employs laser energy in direct contact with adipose tissue to induce lipolysis and, at the same time, coagulate tiny blood vessels and stimulate dermal and subdermal neocollagenesis. These features of laser lipolysis permit a fast, comfortable postoperative recovery, a rapid return to activities of daily living, and excellent skin redraping as a result of laser-induced skin tightening.

THE CLINICS ARE NOW AVAILABLE ONLINE!

Access your subscription at:
www.theclinics.com

Preface
Plastic and Reconstructive Surgery, Ambulatory and Inpatient

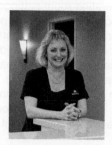

Deborah S. Hickman Mathis, RN, MS, CNOR, RNFA
Guest Editor

Plastic and reconstructive surgery, wound, and hand continue to be the focus of plastic surgery practices, plastic and reconstructive surgery centers, acute care departmental entities, as well as some nontraditional cosmetic spas/facilities. Plastic and reconstructive surgery will affect most people at some point in their or their loved ones' lives. This specialty serves all areas of the body ranging from cosmetic, to restorative, corrective, and functional, to multidisciplinary collaborative procedures. It is the purpose of this issue of *Perioperative Nursing Clinics* to address a few of the many topics facing those in the practice of plastic and reconstructive surgery and those interdepartmental entities that serve the patient collaboratively for the best outcome possible in the provision of their health care. Below, you will find the names, contact information, and mission statements of some of the professional organizations that support the provision of plastic and reconstructive professional practice.

The mission statement of the American Board of Plastic Surgery, Inc (based in Philadelphia, PA, USA; https://www.abplsurg.org/moddefault.aspx) is to promote safe, ethical, efficacious plastic surgery to the public by maintaining high standards for the education, examination, certification, and maintenance of certification of plastic surgeons as specialists and subspecialists.

The American Society for Aesthetic Plastic Surgery (ASAPS), founded in 1967, is the leading professional organization of plastic surgeons certified by the American Board of Plastic Surgery who specializes in cosmetic plastic surgery. With 2600 members in the United States, Canada, and many other countries, ASAPS is at the forefront of innovation in aesthetic plastic surgery around the world (http://www.plasticsurgery. org/). The mission of ASAPS is to advance quality care to plastic surgery patients by encouraging high standards of training, ethics, physician practice, and research in plastic surgery. The society advocates for patient safety, such as requiring its

Perioperative Nursing Clinics 6 (2011) ix–xi
doi:10.1016/j.cpen.2011.04.004
1556-7931/11/$ – see front matter © 2011 Elsevier Inc. All rights reserved.

members to operate in accredited surgical facilities that have passed rigorous external review of equipment and staffing. The society works in concert with the Plastic Surgery Foundation, founded in 1948, that supports research, international volunteer programs, and visiting professor programs.

The American Society of Plastic Surgical Nurses (ASPSN) (https://www.aspsn.org/about.html) was incorporated as a nonprofit organization in 1975. Plastic surgical nursing is a diverse multidisciplinary field that encompasses various practice settings and educational backgrounds, including pediatric reconstruction, skin care, aesthetics, burns, adult reconstruction, craniofacial surgery, operating room settings, postanesthesia care, office settings, management, nurse injectors, independent practitioners, advanced practice nursing, nurse educators, physician assistants, surgical technicians, licensed practical nurses, and industry. The mission of ASPSN is to use education and research to promote practice excellence, nursing leadership, optimal patient safety, and outcomes by using evidence-based practice as a foundation of care.

Cosmetic plastic surgery is safely performed in an accredited office-based surgery facility or freestanding ambulatory surgery facility, or it may be performed in the hospital. When considering surgery, surgeon, and facility, it is important to consider the following and other resources as listed:

Check	Description	How to Check
Board Certification	Certification by an American Board of Medical Specialties (ABMS)– recognized board that is appropriate to the procedure. American Board of Plastic Surgery (ABPS) certification ensures in-depth plastic surgical training.	ABPS: 215.587.9322 or www.abplsurg.org ABMS: www.abms.org
Hospital Privileges	Regardless of where the surgery is to be performed, the surgeon should have privileges to perform the procedure in an acute care hospital.	Ask the professional staff office at the hospital to verify staff privileges.
Surgeon's Experience	An ASAPS membership means a surgeon is ABPS-certified and has significant experience in cosmetic surgery of the face and body.	ASAPS: 888.272.7711 or www.surgery.org
Surgical Facility Accreditation	Facilities should be accredited by a recognized accrediting body, or be state licensed or Medicare certified.	AAAASF: 847.949.6058 or www.aaaasf.org AAAHC: 847.853.6060 or www.aaahc.org JCAHO: 630.792.5000 or www.jcaho.org Check with ndividual states for license information.
Details of Your Surgery	To be discussed before surgery: your complete medical history including past and current medications; surgical benefits, risks, and alternatives; total cost including surgeon fees, anesthesia, facility, and others; surgeon's policy on revisionary procedures; postsurgical care; and typical time line for resuming work/social activities.	Ask your board-certified plastic surgeon

Lastly, I appreciate the efforts of all of the investigators for their contribution, time, and efforts to offer well-presented information for this issue. To all of the readers, I hope this issue will provide you with information, as well as an appetite for plastic, reconstructive, cosmetic, and hand surgeries and related fields.

Deborah S. Hickman Mathis, RN, MS, CNOR, RNFA
Renue Plastic Surgery, Renue Surgery Center
2500 Starling Street, Suite 604
Brunswick, GA 31520, USA

E-mail address:
debbie@renuemd.com

Lastly, I appreciate the efforts of all of the investigators for their contribution, time, and efforts to offer well presented information for this issue. To all of the readers, I hope this issue will provide you with information, as well as an appetite for plastic, reconstructive, cosmetic, and hand surgeries and related fields.

Deborah S. Richman Mathis, RN, MS, CNOR, RNFA
Renue Plastic Surgery, Renue Surgery Center
2500 Starling Street, Suite 604
Brunswick, GA 31520, USA

E-mail address:
debbie@renuernand.com

The Role of Distractions and Interruptions in Operating Room Safety

Theresa (Tess) M. Pape, PhD, RN, CNOR

KEYWORDS

- Operating room safety • Distractions • Interruptions
- Human factors • Culture • Crew resource management
- Teamwork • Signs

Typically, the operating room setting is predisposed to a multitude of distractions leading to a potential for errors. Distractions, lack of focus, poor communication, and not establishing or following standard procedures often lead to problems within any setting.[1]

Certainly, the 1999 Institute of Medicine (IOM) report sounded a sentinel alarm about medical errors in the United States. Its report of approximately 98,000 hospital deaths occurring in US hospitals annually as a result of medical errors led to increased efforts at resolving system problems. Yet little progress has been made in preventing errors.[2] There is a need to reduce errors by improving focus, by using teamwork, decision support, checklists, and other strategies exemplified by other industries such as the aviation industry.[3] Specific conditions within the operating room workplace could be addressed to improve focus and help prevent system errors. "Systems" is a word that is broadly used but often not understood. An explanation of the basics of what makes up a system and how they work together may clarify.

OPEN SYSTEMS

A system is a thing or an organization with interacting parts and subparts. Open systems theory is often used to diagnose system problems by looking at inputs, throughputs, and outputs. Health care organizations typically have open systems, because there are many department entities that interact with each other and with the outside world.[4] Examples of operating room inputs are the characteristics and

Texas Woman's University College of Nursing, PO Box 425498, Denton, TX 76204-5498, USA
E-mail address: tpape10@gmail.com

Perioperative Nursing Clinics 6 (2011) 101–111
doi:10.1016/j.cpen.2011.03.001
1556-7931/11/$ – see front matter © 2011 Published by Elsevier Inc.

periopnursing.theclinics.com

contributions of the perioperative nurses, technicians, physicians, patients, and tools involved in the surgical procedure. Throughputs are the system processes, organizational behavior, and patterns of interaction within the department. The output is the success of the service provided to the patient.[5]

The open system of the operating room is understandably in a constant state of flux in an attempt to balance the environment with organizational goals (**Fig. 1**). System problems hinder the process of getting things done. Once the problem areas are identified, interventions can be developed that resolve the most apparent and frequently occurring problems.[6] In other words, identify the low hanging fruit and pick it first. These are also the areas that could be affected most easily and with lower-cost techniques.

Group processes as a part of throughput include group members' problem-solving techniques and collective beliefs and expectations. People in a group often choose to assist others only after seeking approval from peers, especially when it pertains to safety. However, education provides reasons and principles for changing behavior. Essentially people will listen and abide by rules when provided with rationale for the conduct.[7] To that end, the perioperative nurse plays a key function as a role model in supporting the entire team.

ROLES AND FUNCTIONS IN THE OPERATING ROOM

Operating room settings are very demanding open systems that lend themselves to errors due to the nature of the environment and the fact that people are not perfect. Typically the staff skill mix and experience levels vary greatly, and there are numerous and complex functions expected of each person. Technological equipment and procedures are constantly evolving.[1]

The role of the perioperative nurse as patient advocate requires the nurse to be especially vigilant in terms of patient safety. Although this is expected of perioperative nurses, the ability to remain vigilant is difficult even in the best of circumstances.[8] Typically, patients are interviewed, transported, and transferred many times throughout the process. They come into contact with many medical personnel who perform various technical procedures on them before and during their operative procedure. These multiple points of contact provide numerous opportunities for distractions, interruptions, errors, and misunderstandings of all kinds. Thus, a basic understanding of these factors affecting people can provide insight into error prevention strategies.

HUMAN FACTORS AND ACTIVE FAILURES

The science of understanding human abilities and the effects of outside influences is termed human factors science. This involves all aspects of the way people relate to the organization where they work, with the aim of improving operational performance and safety. Today, health care organizations have become high-reliability organizations in that even though they make mistakes, they also have come to realize that people are humans and that the organization must be constantly preoccupied with the potential for error to occur and prepare in advance. In an ideal world the health care organization as a system has certain defenses or checks and balances that prevent error. However in reality these defenses are like walls of Swiss cheese, and when the holes in the cheese (active and latent failures) line up, mistakes are likely to happen.[9] Distractions, interruptions, and miscommunications are some of the things that can get through the holes.[10]

Active failures are unsafe actions that originate from simply being human. There are limits that can be placed on human cognitive functions and the degree of stimulus that

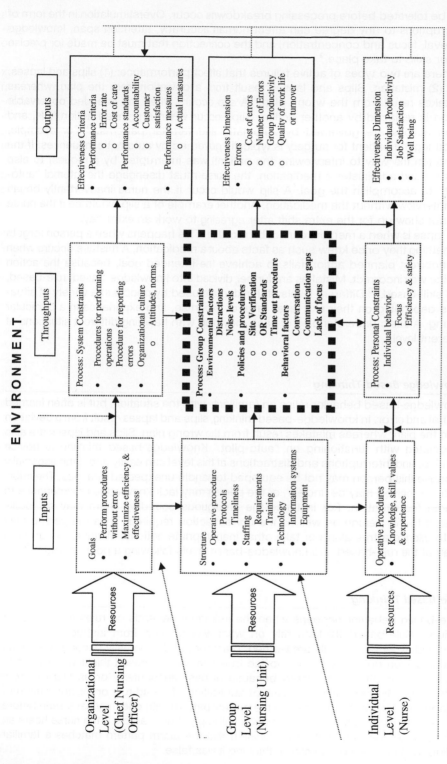

Fig. 1. Operating room safety in hospitals: an organizational framework. (*Data from* Pape TM. Applying airline safety practices to medication administration. Medsurg Nurs 2003;12(2):77–93.)

can be tolerated before processing breakdowns occur. Overstimulation in the form of interruptions to any degree can affect human accuracy, attention span, knowledge retrieval, focus and concentration, and the connection that must be made for precise motor skills to take place.[9]

There are two types of active failures that affect performance: (1) slips and lapses, and (2) mistakes. Slips and lapses result from a deviation from the plan, whereas mistakes result from the wrong plan.[9] A slip occurs when the intended observable action is replaced by another action. Slips occur when a planned action fails, and when actions are governed by automatic and familiar patterns.[10] For example, preparing the patient for surgery is typically governed by automatic influences. If the nurse (on the way to interviewing the patient) was interrupted by a request to also pick up and administer a medication, the nurse must disengage the internal "auto-pilot" to accomplish the goal. A slip would occur if the nurse inadvertently began the interview without the medication. Another example of a slip would be if the nurse did not show up for the extra shift after agreeing to work an extra day.

A lapse is when a memory cannot be recalled. This happens when a person forgets something they once knew such as facts about a medication. A mistake occurs when an incorrect planned action fails to achieve the intended goal, because the action choice was incorrect. Mistakes are further divided into knowledge-based, rule-based, and skill-based.[10] Different levels of thinking are used by people in a variety of situations depending on their skill level, level of expertise, and experience in a particular setting. A basic understanding of each may help with handling different situations at different levels.

Knowledge Based Thinking

Knowledge-based behavior relies on familiarity with the situation, but is often learned by trial and error. In knowledge-based thinking, slips and lapses result from a deviation from the plan, whereas mistakes result from the wrong plan. Slips and lapses are also associated with functioning on "auto-pilot." Knowledge-based thinking is novice thinking, and interruptions and distractions at this level can easily affect the especially because this person may not be equipped to handle unexpected changes. The information received may be unclear, or the person may lack knowledge or experience to handle the situation. For instance the ambiguous sounding alarm may be totally foreign to the person as well as the correct action required. Thus the person may try to silence a true alarm or take other inappropriate actions. Mistakes occur more often at the rule-based and knowledge-based levels following a poor decision.[10]

Rule Based Thinking

Rule-based behavior happens when the individual depends on rules to guide their actions. Rule-based thinkers rely on what was learned from instruction or from personal experience. Skills are learned, practiced, and eventually become automatic as the person progresses from novice to expert. In rule-based thinking, changes in situations are often anticipated because of past encounters, or as learned from instructors. Mistakes arise because of application of a bad rule or misapplication of a good rule. People tend to match the current pattern with one they have seen before and tend to think that the same solution will apply. For example if the nurse hears an alarm, he or she may make the decision that the alarm pattern matches a familiar sound, and ignore the true alarm, thinking it was false.[10]

Skill Based Thinking

With skill based thinking, the character and timing of the change may be known, but an alternate choice has not been fully planned. Slips result primarily from failures on the skill-based level. Though the chances for errors at this level are usually less, they have a greater magnitude of inaccuracy (strong-but-wrong).[10] An example would be in the case of an experienced circulating nurse who forgets to provide clear instructions when relieved for lunch by a novice nurse. While busy with another task the novice nurse failed to act when hearing an alarm he or she had never heard before. The results could be problematic for many involved. **Fig. 2** summarizes distinctions between skill-based, rule-based, and knowledge-based errors and their potential failure mode. Errors at any of the three levels vary depending on cognitive limits placed on a person such as interruptions, distractions, and preoccupations, and the type of task involved.

Short and Long Term Memory

Short term and long term memory play a part in errors as well. Indeed active failures (slips, memory lapses) affect the short term memory. The short term or working memory is used for attention, consciousness, and the storage of small amounts of information such as remembering a list of three items without writing them down.[9] Active failures can result when sharp attention or alertness is required, but for which the elements for this heightened alertness were not provided. Humans cannot remain alert for more than 10 to 20 minutes when expected to watch for rare events.[10] For example, perioperative nurses must maintain vigilance over: the sterility of the procedure, the proper sequencing of events, the status of the patient, and the accuracy of documentation. Any interruption or distraction can jeopardize this vigilance. This leads to a discussion of the rationale for considering latent conditions.

HUMAN FACTORS AND LATENT FAILURES

Latent failures are those things that contribute to error from outside the person or allow interference to continue. Environmental pressures, noise, and interruptions of activity can cause omitted actions when the intended action is lost due to the delay between forming the thought and the time it takes to complete the action. Redirection becomes even more difficult when the interruption was unrelated to the current action being performed.[10]

The Operating Room Environment

The operating room environment is an example of a complex system with the potential for multiple latent conditions affecting the nurse's capacity to maintain alertness, vigilance, critical thinking, and good decision making. Latent conditions (distractions, interruptions, time pressures, and noise) are linked to conditions within the work environment. When latent failures combine with active failures, mistakes are more likely to happen. As a result, interruptions can cause a loss of focus at a critical time that can be hazardous. Excessive input (information overload), and interruptions and distractions compete for attention and fill the working memory where information is temporarily stored, thus affecting the ability to concentrate.[9]

The person initiating an interruption often uses a physical signal of some kind, and that signal passes a detection threshold of the recipient's senses, causing the recipient to respond. Recipients of interruptions take the role of accepting the interruption, and are usually expected to attend to another task as a result. The success of the interruption depends on the recipient's threshold and acceptance of the interference. In a recent study medical doctors and registered nurses in an emergency department

FACTOR	Skill-Based Errors	Rule-Based Errors	Knowledge-Based Errors
Type of Activity	Routine actions	Problem-solving actions	
Focus of Attention	On other things than the task.	Directed at problem-related issues.	
Control Mode	Affect automatic processors (action plan)	(stored rules)	Limited conscious processes.
Predictability of Error Type.	Largely predictable "strong but wrong" errors.		Variable
Ratio of Error to Opportunity for Error.	Constitutes a small proportion of total number of chances for error.		
Situational Influence	Low to moderate; internal factors & prior experience likely to influence.		External factors dominate.
Ease of Detection	Detection usually rapid and effective.	Difficult and often only achieved through external intervention.	
Relationship to Change	Knowledge of change not accessed at proper time.	When and how anticipated change will occur is unknown.	Changes not prepared for or anticipated.
Failure Modes & Error Potentials	**Inattention** Slips, Omissions after interruptions or distractions. Easily distracted. Perceptual confusions. Interference errors. **Overattention** Omissions Repetitions Reversals	**Misapplication of good rules** Mistakes Information overload. **Bad rules applied** Mistakes Encoding deficie Action deficiency Wrong rules. Bad rules.	**Mistakes Caused By** Workspace limitations. Out of sight out of mind. Confirmation bias. Overconfidence. Biased reviewing. Halo effects Causality problems. Complexity problems.

Fig. 2. Distinctions between skill-based, rule-based, and knowledge-based errors. (*Data from* Reason J. Human error. New York: Cambridge University Press; 1990.)

were observed in their role of being the initiator or the recipient of interruptions. Registered nurses were more likely to accept interruptions than were physicians. Medical doctors received 10.58 interruptions per hour compared with 11.65 times per hour for registered nurses. Registered nurses tended to initiate interruptions with other registered nurses more than with medical doctors. However, medical doctors received an interruption more often than they initiated an interruption. Similarly, registered nurses initiated an interruption less often than they accepted interruptions. The study suggests that there is a need for more research to determine why interruptions are initiated and received, and that there is a need to design effective strategies to reduce interruptions.[11] Periopertive nurses should consider whether they may have tendencies to accept or initiate interruptions, and consider what strategies could be taken to lessen them.

People can make errors in any situation, but the high risk hectic nature of most operating room settings provide a greater potential for mistakes. The current shortage of perioperative nurses offers more opportunities for increased errors as operating room departments try to do more with fewer nurses. In an effort to maintain the operative schedule, personnel often become hurried, distracted, and interrupted during critical steps in a process. In such systems there is little ability to predict problems before they occur. Nevertheless, a look at the role of interruptions and distractions on those who work in the operating room can offer insight into solutions.

Distractions and Interruptions

Distractions and interruptions including noise and conversation are constraints affecting the operating room system that can lead to errors. The operating room can be a very noisy setting with conversations occurring simultaneously in crowded spaces. Many operating rooms settings allow the playing of music, which can often be distracting. Nurses frequently perform more than 1 task at a time within this noisy and complicated setting. For example, they often take phone calls while performing sponge counts and charting, and may then be interrupted by someone entering the room to speak with the surgeon or ask a question.

According to research findings, leading factors contributing to medication errors are poor lighting, distractions, interruptions, multitasking, hurriedness, and the effects of fatigue. Distractions include any action that draws away, diverts, or disturbs the mind or attention from achieving a goal and are a leading cause of errors. One study found that distraction-reducing interventions are effective strategies that can affect systems within the hospital setting, and have the potential to reduce errors. The study evaluated the effectiveness of focused protocols and teamwork to decrease distractions and interruptions. Results indicate that distractions can be significantly reduced by educating staff members of the importance of others not distracting nurses during critical times. In addition, nurses' avoidance of extraneous conversation and use of visible signage provided more reduction in distractions.[12] Thus, it stands to reason that medication errors and other types of errors could be reduced by decreasing distractions and interruptions in the operating room setting.

Organizational Culture and Safety

Culture is a set of norms, attitudes, and values inherent within the organization defined by the importance placed on the work done. The organizational structure involves relations between individuals, groups, and positions. Organizational culture shapes the work, the change process, the power held by others, and the impact of external trends.[4] Certainly management places constraints on organizational culture in many ways. Managers create the qualities of organizational culture when ranking objectives in terms of safety, profit, service, values, and operating standards. Such shaping may be deliberate or accidental, depending on financial constraints and value systems, and whether the managerial culture supports learning from past errors. Those in administration also exercise control over safety by the type of equipment purchased, staffing levels, patterns of shift work, and bonuses for good work or sanctions for bad work.[7] If safety and error prevention, innovation, and teamwork are not valued by managers, they will not be valued among perioperative staff either. When managers are not perceived as concerned about safety, employees will follow with the same attitude. Further, if employees do not trust management, they will reject any new safety initiatives. Effective changes begin with management that supports a safety culture by walking the walk of safety not just by talking the talk. When new employees come aboard, someone who exemplifies the safety culture should mentor them.[13] Ultimately organizational culture either supports or detracts from organizational effectiveness. Teamwork has also been an important contributor in assisting nurses to avoid distractions.[14]

Team Problems

Team structures often lose cohesiveness as constraints from social dynamics can cause them to become an informal group. Subsequently, when a formal authority structure is lacking, the team functions ineffectively. Even if some in the team remain efficient, social pressures by other team members eventually cause behavior conformity. Teams lose functionality when there is a lack of leadership, failure to follow rules of operation, and when members become too informal with each other, and allow peer pressure to affect appropriate behavior and choices.[7]

The airplane cockpit demonstrates one example of the importance of teamwork, with clear lines of authority and effective communication. Pilots follow standard operating procedures and checklists that direct their actions. Nevertheless, changes can occur that require coordinated efforts between all team members. Airline research finds that errors take place most often because of failures in teamwork and coordination. Complex work such as that involved in the operating room also requires teamwork. Thus, following the example of the aviation industry by training teams to work harmoniously can improve safety.[13,14] Leaders must demonstrate support for safety and expect their employees to model an attitude of safety in all work relations.

Noise pollution in the operating room has a cumulative effect that hinders caregivers' abilities to perform their jobs and to hear their colleagues clearly. Although perioperative staff members usually learn to cope with the noise pollution by elevating their voices, compromised hearing can lead to adverse patient outcomes. Reducing noise as a distraction in the operating room is recognized as an important function of the team, especially during critical times such as during the time out procedure and during patient anesthesia induction and emergence. A wrong site surgery was performed at Beth Israel Deaconess Medical Center in Boston in 2008 when the surgical team failed to correctly hear the verification of the procedure due to noise. Increasing staff awareness of the role of noise can also help reduce errors involving sound alike medications.[15] Today, many operating room departments may have become complacent to the importance of focus and concentration on error prevention. Streams of visitors, students, and parents are often allowed in the operating area at inopportune times. There is a scarcity of interventions addressing human factors and work redesign that have been applied to reduce errors in the operating room.

PROPOSED SOLUTIONS

The solution for high-reliability organizations such as health care is to bullet proof the safety system as much as possible in spite of human and organizational hazards. No matter how effective the system, there will always be setbacks and errors. What is important is that learning from errors occurs and corrective actions are taken that provide additional resilience for the future. Nevertheless, health care should apply safety techniques found in the airline and other high-reliability industries.[8,14] A desired situation in any operating room suite would be to have as few distractions and interruptions as possible, to reduce noise levels, and improve teamwork.

In terms of human factor approaches, those who operate at the knowledge-based, rule-based, and skill-based levels need specific strategies to avoid errors.[9] Innovative methods that reduce distractions and interruptions, and promote focus and attention are needed to help prevent errors. Process changes could be implemented without undue hardship. Many are simple and inexpensive, and error prevention would result. In addition staff members would likely benefit from decreases in confusion in the operating room environment. Nevertheless, implementing solutions to distraction, interruption, noise, and communication problems in any environment can pose challenges.

Protocols and Visible Signage

The world of symbols, values, social entities, and cultures is something very important to people. People have increasingly become symbol-making, symbol-using, symbol-dominated creatures.[16] Signs can serve as warning of impending danger or error messages before the fact.[9] Signs are also useful reminders of the priority of safety and act as activators to direct behavior.[7] For example, signs can be used in the operating room so that others recognize a heightened awareness of risk. Signs can be used as reminders not to distract or interrupt during critical times.

Because noise is an increased stressor, one New York hospital used several interventions including "Shhh" signs to reduce conversation and noise as distracters. Before implementation of the program, noise levels were 90 to 115 decibels, but afterward they decreased to an average of 57.5 decibels.[17]

One phenomenon often encountered with signage is habituation or ignoring a sign or sound. This is important so one can ignore fairly innocuous distractions such as billboards while driving. However, the importance of having a safe environment increases the potential for continued compliance. People who believe that the safety goal is worthwhile, and that the consequences are unacceptable, will abide by the signs.[7] Decreasing the potential for error provides a worthwhile safety incentive to abide by signs and reduce distractions and interruptions.

Team Approaches

When all team members feel respected and valued, and hierarchies are eliminated, communication patterns can improve and distractions be reduced. Such an environment helps reduce communication problems that can lead to interruptions. Situational awareness is also needed so the operating room team knows when reduced communication is appropriate as well as when to speak up.[1]

A recent study found that the use of teamwork approaches borrowed from the aviation industry in the form of crew resource management reduced surgical instrument and needle count errors by 50%. Attitudes were changed about the value of teamwork to reduce errors. Processes were standardized with checklists, and team communication skills improved.[18] Likewise, other standardizations can be effective at improving team function and reducing distractions.

Because the open system of the operating room setting is in a constant state of flux, standard operating procedures must be addressed (see **Fig. 1**). The system group level is the most likely area for improvements in throughput (bolded area in **Fig. 1**), and is most logical for addressing interruptions, distractions, and improving teamwork.

The Association of Perioperative Nurses (AORN) continually supports a noise-controlled environment and one that reduces interruptions and distractions. Some of the AORN's suggestions include:

Identifying sources of noise in the operating room so they can be reduced
Brainstorming to develop strategies to control noise
Leaving personal cell phones and pagers out of the operating room setting
Limiting essential phone conversations, muting nonessential devices
Controlling one's own voice tone
Limiting or toning down music playing
Using building supplies that reduce noise during renovation
Setting monitor noise levels appropriately
Replacing noisy metal carts with quiet ones (perhaps plastic)
Encouraging research and development on noise reduction strategies
Increasing staff awareness about reducing noise
Limiting the number of people in the operating room
Limiting overhead paging
Displaying "Quiet, Please" posters.[19]

Other potential solutions to reduce interruptions and distractions include:

Using visible signage such as "Operative Procedure in Progress—Do Not Disturb" outside of each operating room
Holding up or posting a "SHHH" sign during anesthesia induction and emergence
Educating staff members about the importance of reducing interruptions
Establishing a sterile cockpit atmosphere during critical times in which no unnecessary conversation is acceptable
Reducing noise levels of all kinds
Promoting teamwork and effective communication
Redesigning the workflow to improve processes and reduce interruptions
Identifying and limiting tendencies to accept or initiate interruptions.

SUMMARY

Today, perioperative nurses are under increasing pressures almost daily, and there are numerous and complex functions expected of each person. Operating room settings are very demanding open systems that lend themselves to errors. System problems are constraints to getting things done. These include breakdowns in both work design and environmental design. Design failures involve problems with process, tasks, or equipment. System failures include high noise levels, distractions, interruptions, ineffective communication, lack of focus, and lack of teamwork.

Safety within the operating room begins with strong leadership and management principles. Employees will follow the attitude and policies emulated by those in administrative roles. It is time for innovative strategies to reduce interruptions and prevent errors in the operative environment. Several evidence-based strategies borrowed from aviation can prevent errors. These include posting of signs as effective reminders of the priority of safety and to act as activators to direct behavior. Checklist protocols should also be used to reduce distractions and interruptions within the operating room department. Ultimately, redesigning operating room work processes is vital to helping people avoid errors and their consequences.

REFERENCES

1. Miller K, editor. Safety in the operating room: improving healthcare quality and safety. Joint Commission; 2006.
2. Institute of Medicine Committee. In: Kohn LT, Corrigan JM, Donaldson MS, editors. To err is human: building a safer health system. Washington, DC: National Academy Press; 2000.
3. Agency for Healthcare Research and Quality. Evidence report/technology assessment: making health care safer: a critical analysis of patient safety practices summary. 2001. Available at: http://archive.ahrq.gov/clinic/ptsafety/pdf/front.pdf. Accessed January 14, 2011.
4. Harrison MI, Shirom A. Organizational diagnosis and assessment: bridging theory and practice. Thousand Oaks (CA): Sage; 1999.
5. Pape TM. The effect of nurses' use of a focused protocol to decrease distractions during medication administration [published doctoral dissertation]. Denton (TX): Texas Woman's University, College of Nursing; 2002.
6. Goldratt EM. Critical chain. Great Barrington (MA): North River Press; 1997.
7. Geller ES. The psychology of safety handbook. Boca Raton (FL): Lewis Publishers; 2001.
8. Moray N. Error reduction as a systems problem. In: Bogner MS, editor. Human error in medicine. Hillsdale (NJ): Erlbaum Associates; 1994. p. 67–91.
9. Reason J. Human error: models and management. BMJ 2000;320(7237):768–70.
10. Reason J. Human error. New York: Cambridge University Press; 1990.
11. Brixey JJ, Robinson DJ, Turley JP, Zhang J. Initiators of interruption in workflow: the role of MDs and RNs. Stud Health Technol Inform 2007;130:103–39.
12. United States Pharmacopeia. Physical environments that promotes safe medication use. 2010. Available at: http://www.usp.org/pdf/EN/USPNF/gc1066Physical Environments.pdf. Accessed January 10, 2011.
13. Helmreich RL, Merritt AC. Culture at work in aviation and medicine: National, organizational and professional influences. Brookfield (VT): Ashgate Publishing; 1998.
14. Sculli GL, Sine DM. Soaring to success: taking crew resource management from the cockpit to the nursing unit. Philadelphia: HCPro, Inc; 2011.
15. Stanton C. Controlling noise in the OR. AORN Connections; 2009.
16. Von Bertalanffy L. Robots, men and minds: psychology in the modern world. New York: George Brazilier; 1967.
17. Montefore Medical Center. Silent hospitals help healing. Available at: http://www.montefiore.org/whoweare/stories/shhh/. Accessed January 10, 2011.
18. Rivers RM, Swain D, Nixon WR. Using aviation safety measures to enhance patient outcomes. AORN J 2003;77:158–62.
19. Aorn. AORN's position statement on noise in the perioperative setting. 2009. Available at: http://www.aorn.org/PracticeResources/AORNPositionStatements/PositionStatementOnNoise/. Accessed January 12, 2011.

Skin Antisepsis: First Line of Defense Set Skin Preparation in Motion Before the Incision

Judith Seltzer, MS, BSN, RN, CNOR

KEYWORDS

- Skin preparation agents • Manufacturer's instructions
- Surgical-site infection • Antiseptic agents

In 1992 the US Centers for Disease Control (CDC) revised its definition of wound infection, creating the definition surgical-site infection (SSI). SSIs are infections that occur at any site along the surgical tract.[1]

Prevention of SSIs continues to be one of the greatest health care challenges in the world today. It is estimated that, in the United States alone, there are some 27 million annual surgical procedures resulting in 500,000 surgical-site infections.[2] These infections have proved to be a major cause of patient injury and mortality, as well as adding to ever-increasing health care costs. Overall, SSIs are associated with $7 billion to $10 billion annually. In health care expenditures in the United States:

- An estimated 2.6% of nearly 30 million operations are complicated by SSIs each year
- Infection rates of up to 11% are reported for certain types of operations
- Each infection is estimated to increase a hospital stay by an average of 7 days and add more than $3000 in charges (1992 data).[3]

The patient's own indigenous flora is the most common form of pathogen transmission leading to an SSI.[4] Therefore, once the surgical incision has been made, the patient's skin is no longer intact and is at risk for an infection to occur. Therefore, preparing the patients skin before the incision is made can potentially the patient from developing a SSI. The CDC defines surgical skin preparation as a "procedure for cleansing the skin with an antiseptic before the surgical procedure."[1] In the CDC Surgical-Site Infection Guidelines (1999), requiring patients to shower or bathe with an antiseptic agent on at least the night before the operative day is listed as a category

Molnlycke Health Care, 2611 Fallston Road, Fallston, MD 21047, USA
E-mail address: judith.seltzer@molnlycke.com

Perioperative Nursing Clinics 6 (2011) 113–124
doi:10.1016/j.cpen.2011.03.002

Box 1
CDC Recommended Guidelines rationale

Category 1A

Strongly recommended for implementation and supported by well-designed experimental, clinical, or epidemiologic studies

Category IB

Strongly recommended for implementation and supported by some experimental, clinical, or epidemiologic studies and strong theoretic rationale

Category II

Suggested for implementation and supported by suggestive clinical or epidemiologic studies or theoretic rationale

No recommendation (unresolved issue)

Practices for which insufficient evidence or no consensus regarding efficacy exists

Adapted from Appendix J. CDC Recommendation for the prevention of surgical site infections. 1999 Adapted from Mangram, HICPAC and CDC. Available at: http://www.cec.gov/ncidod/hip/SSI/SSI_guideline.htm.

IB recommendation (**Box 1**).[1] It is strongly recommended that all surgical patients receive preoperative skin cleansing before their procedure, regardless of surgery type.

According to the Association of periOperative Registered Nurses (AORN)
Recommended practice for preoperative patient skin antisepsis,[5] the goal of the skin preparation process is to:
- Reduce the risk of surgical-site infections by removing soil and transient organisms from the patient's skin
- Reduce the resident microbial count in a short period of time
- Inhibit rebound growth of microorganisms
- Be performed in a manner that preserves skin integrity and prevents injury to the skin.

Rationale:
- Important factors to consider regarding surgical skin preparation outcomes include removal of pathogens while preserving skin integrity.

US FOOD AND DRUG ADMINISTRATION REGULATIONS OF ANTISEPTICS

In the United States, drugs, pharmaceuticals, and cosmetics are regulated by the Food and Drug Administration (FDA). Thus antiseptics are under the jurisdiction of, and have parameters clearly defined by, the FDA. The health care facility should use FDA-approved agents that have immediate, cumulative, and persistent antimicrobial action[6]:

- The skin preparation agents should have the following properties: fast-acting, persistent and cumulative, and nonirritating
- The surgical team members and infection prevention practitioner should be involved in the process of evaluating and selecting the skin preparation agents. In the United States, antiseptic agents are regulated by the FDA's Division of Over-the-Counter Drug Products[5]

- The evaluation should involve the review of the manufacturer's information to confirm that the antiseptic agents were tested according to FDA requirements and to review the results of the testing to confirm efficacy of the product.

The involvement of the surgical personnel allows the evaluation of the properties of the antiseptic agents, including effects on the skin, and contributes to the final decision regarding the antiseptic agents that are the most effective antimicrobial solutions as well as least harmful to the skin.

When evaluating antiseptic agents, the following FDA standards should be taken into consideration. The agents should substantially reduce transient microorganisms; possess a broad spectrum of antimicrobial properties; be fast acting; have persistent, cumulative activity; and be nonirritating to the skin.[5]

MOST FREQUENTLY USED SKIN PREPARATION AGENTS

Plastic, cosmetic, and reconstructive surgery refers to a variety of operations performed to repair or restore body parts to look normal, or to change a body part to look better. These types of surgery are highly specialized. They are characterized by careful preparation of the patient's skin and tissues, by precise cutting and suturing techniques, and by care taken to minimize scarring.

The risks associated with plastic, cosmetic, and reconstructive surgery include the postoperative complications that can occur with any surgical procedure. However, these types of surgical procedures also carry specific risks for the patient:

- Formation of undesirable scar tissue
- Persistent pain, redness, or swelling in the area of the surgery
- Infection inside the body related to insertion of a prosthesis. These infections can result from contamination at the time of surgery or from bacteria migrating into the area around the prosthesis at a later time.

But when it comes to surgical skin preparation, plastic surgery is no different from other service lines. Patients must be protected from developing SSI's. The 1999 CDC SSI guidelines require the "use of an appropriate agent for skin preparation."[1] These guidelines discuss several skin preparation agents that are in use today. Currently, the 2 most common skin preparation agents used in plastic/reconstructive surgery are chlorhexidine gluconate (CHG), (with or without alcohol), and povidone-iodine (with or without alcohol) (**Table 1**).[7]

According to the CDC, some comparisons of the 2 antiseptics when used as preoperative hand scrubs suggest that chlorhexidine gluconate achieved greater reductions in skin microflora than did povidone-iodine and also had greater residual activity after a single application.[1] When reviewing literature of skin preparation agents, more and more researchers/practitioners are concluding that CHG is superior to other products related to skin disinfection. In a study by Darouiche and colleagues,[8] preoperative cleansing of the patient's skin with chlorhexidine-alcohol is superior to cleansing with povidone-iodine for preventing SSI after clean contaminated surgery. In a separate study by Fletcher and colleagues,[9] chlorhexidine gluconate was found to be superior to povidone-iodine for preoperative antisepsis for both the patient and surgeon.

The major caveat to these and similar studies was that, although the best outcomes were achieved using CHG, the CHG was combined with alcohol. Alcohol is flammable product.

In an article by Prasad and colleagues,[10] the use of alcohol-based products for hand hygiene and skin antisepsis could initiate even greater concerns regarding the hazards

Table 1
Characteristics of CHG, povidone-iodine, and alcohol

Agent	Activity	Characteristics	Efficacy	Indications
CHG	Disruption of cytoplasmic membranes Binds to the corneum stratum	Broad spectrum Considered nontoxic Not for use past superficial layers of skin Not for use in eyes, ears, and mucous membranes Excellent antiseptic Immediate activity Persistent effect Cumulative effect	Excellent bactericidal Effective against enveloped viruses Activity affected by anionic surfactants	Hand scrubs Hand antisepsis in high-risk areas Skin preparation
Povidone-iodine	Rapidly penetrates cell walls and inactivates cells	Broad spectrum Activity substantially reduced in the presence of organic material (eg, blood) Poor persistent activity	Bactericidal Active against TB, fungi, and viruses	Surgical hand scrubs Skin preparation
Alcohol	Denatures proteins	Excellent germicidal Needs emollients Higher concentrations may lead to higher risk of flammability	Excellent bactericidal Excellent against TB Good virucidal Rapid onset Must be allowed to dry fully No appreciable persistent activity once it has evaporated	Surgical hand scrubs Surgical hand rubs Not recommended for use on soil and debris

Abbreviation: TB, tuberculosis.
Data from Boyce JM, Pittet D. Guideline for hand hygiene in health-care settings. Recommendations of the Healthcare Infection Control Practice Advisory Committee and the HICPAC/SHEA/APIC/IDSA Hand hygiene Task Force. MMWR Recomm Rep 2002;51:1.

of operating room fires. In the case study reviewed in the article by Prasad and colleagues,[10] the patient was scheduled for a tracheostomy.

The surgical site was prepared according to the facility protocol with a 1-step skin preparation agent with an alcohol solution covering the face, neck, shoulders, and upper chest. An oxygen-rich environment was ruled out as a possible cause of the surgical fire. The initial site of fire corresponded with the distribution of skin preparation agent used to prepare the surgical site. In addition, the short time between the preparation of the surgical site and the use of the electrosurgical unit (the ignition source) suggested that the solution in some areas of the surgical field was not yet entirely dry and that the amount of alcohol vapor was substantial. The distribution of the burned area on the patient corresponded with the distribution of the antiseptic solution. It was therefore confirmed in this particular case that the use of an alcohol-based antiseptic was the major contributing factor to the surgical fire.

One could therefore conclude that, based on the literature available today, CHG without the use of alcohol is a beneficial step to promoting the best surgical outcomes for our patients.

TYPES OF SKIN PREPARATION

Although the types of surgery frequently seen are related to the term plastic surgery, advances in the development of miniaturized instruments, new materials for artificial limbs and body parts, and improved surgical techniques have expanded the range of plastic surgery operations that can be performed. Three types of surgery share some common techniques and approaches, even though they have somewhat different emphases.[11]

- Plastic surgery is usually performed to treat birth defects and to remove skin blemishes such as warts, acne scars, or birthmarks
- Cosmetic surgery procedures are performed to make patients look younger or to enhance their appearance in other ways
- Reconstructive surgery is used to reattach body parts severed in combat or accidents, to perform skin grafts after severe burns, or to reconstruct parts of the patient's body that were missing at birth or removed by surgery. Reconstructive surgery is the oldest form of plastic surgery, having developed out of the need to treat wounded soldiers in wartime.

Based on these advances, it is common to see more procedures scheduled using the terminology of plastic surgery (**Box 2**). One can see by the list that implementing a solid surgical skin protocol provides best practice measures to surgical patients since so many areas of the body are now classified as plastic surgery.

SURGICAL SKIN PREPARATION STARTS AT HOME

Only in recent years have protocols been developed that enlist the patient to act as partner in the battle toward reducing SSIs. In today's health care environment, patients are being instructed to cleanse their skin before entering the facility before their procedure. A preoperative shower or bath decreases the microbial count on a patient's skin.

A study by Rao and colleagues[12] in 2008 showed that a preoperative decolonization protocol (which implemented 4% chlorhexidine baths) for staphylococcus infections in patients having total joint arthroplasty translated to an adjusted economic gain of approximately $230,000 to the facility. Patients in the study were instructed to shower or bathe 4 nights before the day of surgery and then shower or bathe on the morning of surgery before entering the facility.

Much of the reason for using a 4% CHG formula is that it bonds directly with the skin, immediately killing existing microbes, and continuing to kill microbes for up to 6 hours. Several applications of CHG help attain maximum antimicrobial benefits, so patients are generally instructed to complete repeated antiseptic baths or showers to achieve expected best outcomes.

In 2008, AORN issued guidelines that recommend the use of body washes that contain 4% CHG for at-home use before surgery, specifically the night before and

> **Box 2**
> **Procedure areas identified for plastic surgery**
>
> 1. Lateral thoracoabdominal preparation
>
>   The area includes axilla, chest, and abdomen from the neck to crest of the ilium. Area extends beyond the midline, anterior and posterior. Patient is in lateral position on the operating table
>
> 2. Abdominal preparation
>
>   The area includes breast line to upper third of thighs, from the table line, with patient in supine position
>
> 3. Chest and breast preparation
>
>   The area includes shoulder, upper arm down to elbow, axilla and chest wall to the table line beyond sternum to opposite shoulder. The patient may be in a lateral position
>
> 4. Knee and Lower leg preparation
>
>   The area includes the entire circumference of affected leg and extends from foot to upper part of thigh
>
> 5. Rectoperineal and vaginal preparation
>
>   The area includes pubis, vulva, labia, perineum, anus, and adjacent areas including inner aspects of upper thigh
>
> 6. Hip preparation
>
>   The area includes the abdomen on the affected side, thigh to the knees, buttock to table line, groin, and pubis
>
> *From* Survey of standard operating room procedures. Sweet Haven Publishing Services. Available at: www.waybuilder.net/./Surgery02. Accessed December 03, 2010; with permission.

the morning of surgery.[5] Sample instructions, although basic, adapted from the American Red Cross, aim to help patients understand the importance as well as the understanding of how to bathe thoroughly (**Box 3**).[13,14]

ON ARRIVAL AT THE FACILITY

A skin preparation protocol should be followed on the patient's arrival to the facility. The preoperative patient interview should include asking patients whether they have completed their 4% CHG skin cleansing protocols as directed by their physicians. In addition, completing a thorough review with the patient will reveal any known allergies that may affect the skin preparation agent that will be used before surgery.

If the information gathered from the interview indicates that the patient is allergic to shellfish and likely has an iodine allergy, a noniodine preparation solution should be used. If the information gathered from the interview indicates that the patient is allergic to CHG, then products containing CHG should not be used.

This information should be recorded on the patient data assessment document to ensure that all information relative to the surgical procedure will be available if the patient contracts a SSI after their surgical procedure.

ASEPTIC TECHNIQUE: ALIVE AND WORKING IN TODAY'S OPERATING ROOM

Before the skin preparation of a patient is initiated, the skin should be free of gross contamination (ie, dirt, soil, or any other debris). The following AORN recommended practices are used daily practice throughout hospitals across the country (**Box 4**).[5]

Box 3
General skin cleansing instructions before surgery

Before you bathe or shower:

- Read the instructions given to you by your health care practitioner. Begin your skin cleansing protocol according to your provider and/or facility instructions
- Carefully read all directions on the product label
- CHG should not be used on the face, including around the eyes and ears
- CHG is not to be used on mucous membranes, including use in genital area
- Do not use product if you are allergic to CHG

During your bath or shower:

- If you plan to wash your hair, do so with your regular shampoo. Then rinse hair and body thoroughly to remove any shampoo residue
- Wash your face with your regular soap or water only
- Thoroughly rinse your body with warm water from the neck down.
- Apply the minimum amount of CHG necessary to cover the skin, using it as you would any other liquid soap, applying it directly on the skin and washing gently
- Rinse thoroughly with warm water
- Do not use your regular soap after applying and rinsing a CHG product
- After rinsing, gently pat skin dry with towel

Morning of surgery and/or procedure

- Shower again using CHG in the same method as described earlier
- Do not apply any lotions, deodorants, powders, or perfumes to the body areas that have been cleansed with CHG

Data from Sorrentino S. Assisting with patient care. St Louis (MO): Mosby; 2006. p. 305–10; and American Red Cross. Modified bed bath, skill 12. State of Maryland; 2009.

The skin around the surgical site should be free of soil, debris, exudates, and transient microorganisms. Cleaning certain areas first reduces bacterial counts (eg, umbilicus).

Safe skin preparation activities include[5]:

- Agents should be applied by nonscrubbed personnel once hand hygiene has been completed
- The health care practitioner should use sterile supplies, including the use of sterile gloves
- As with all skin preparation agents, following the manufacturers instructions is crucial to providing the best care to the patient
- The health care practitioner performing the skin preparation should place protective barriers, beginning at the preparation periphery, to prevent the accumulation of the agent or pooling to avoid chemical burns and skin irritation
- Applying an antiseptic agent in concentric circles, beginning in the area of the proposed incision and moving to the periphery. The prepared area should be large enough to extend the incision or create new incisions or drain sites, if necessary
- The preparation applicator should be used for single applications and then discarded, using a fresh applicator with subsequent applications

Box 4
AORN recommended practices 2010: perioperative patient skin antisepsis

- Recommended Practice I
  - The surgical site and surrounding areas should be clean
- Recommended Practice II
  - The surgical site and surrounding area should be prepared with an antiseptic agent that has been FDA approved
- Recommended Practice III
  - The antiseptic agent should be selected based on the patient assessment
- Recommended Practice IV
  - Whenever possible, hair should be left at the surgical site
- Recommended Practice V
  - The skin around the surgical site should be free of soil and debris
- Recommended Practice VI
  - Protective measures should be in place to preserve skin integrity and prevent injury to the skin
- Recommended Practice VII
  - The antiseptic agent should be placed over the surgical site in a manner that minimizes contamination, preserves skin integrity, and prevents tissue damage
- Recommended Practice VIII
  - If flammable agents are used, protective measures must be taken
- Recommended Practice IX
  - Manufacturers instructions and label directives must be followed
- Recommended Practice X
  - At the end of the procedure, the agent must be removed unless otherwise directed by the manufacturer
- Recommended Practice XI
  - Personnel should maintain competency by completing proper training
- Recommended Practice XII
  - Patient skin preparation should be documented in the patient's record
- Recommended Practice XIII
  - Policies and procedures for the skin preparation should be written, reviewed annually, and easily accessible
- Recommended Practice XIV
  - A quality management program should be in place to evaluate skin preparation methods and agents

From AORN Perioperative Standards and Recommended Practices. RP Preoperative Patient Skin Antisepsis. Denver (CO): the Association of Perioperative Registered Nurses. Copyright © 2009 AORN, Inc; 2010. p. 351–69; with permission.

- When not part of the procedure, highly contaminated sites such as colostomies should be isolated before the application of the skin preparation agent
- On completion of the skin preparation, the health care practitioner removes protective barriers and rechecks the patient for any pooling of antiseptic agents
- At the completion of the surgical procedure, remaining preparation agent should be removed from the patient's skin to avoid postoperative skin irritations.

There are reports of modifications to the procedure according to the location and type of skin preparation needed.[1] Surgical procedures such as grafts may require 2 separate skin preparations to be completed. When prepping donor and recipient sites, the donor site is usually prepped first, allowing for good visualization for the surgeon. Eye and facial preparations may require the use of alternative skin preparation agents. CHG and iodine based alcohol products are contraindicated for the eyes and ears. Because of this, many plastic surgeons elect to use an iodine paint solution for the skin preparation for surgical procedures above the chin. If patients are awake for the procedure, they should be advised to keep their eyes closed and the eyes should be rinsed with warm sterile water if the agent leaks into the eyes. If the patient is allergic to iodine, then plastic surgeons often elect to use sterile water as their agent of choice for the skin preparation.

In an independent survey conducted for this article, 22 plastic surgery teams were surveyed from 9 facilities addressing the following questions:

1. What skin preparation agents do you use for procedures in areas below the chin?
2. What skin preparation agents do you use for procedures above the chin?
3. How do you prepare the skin if the patient is allergic to iodine and/or CHG?

According to the survey results, most of those surveyed prepare the skin for surgeries conducted below the chin with a CHG agent containing alcohol. For procedures above the chin, all teams surveyed stated that skin was prepared with an iodine paint agent. Those surveyed identified that, if the patient was allergic to iodine, sterile water was the agent of choice, because CHG was not indicated for areas around the eyes and ear (**Table 2**).

Table 2
Independent survey of plastic surgeons related to the skin preparation agent used

Agent	Below Chin	Above Chin	Below Chin but Allergic to Iodine	Below Chin but Allergic to CHG	Above Chin but Allergic to Iodine
CHG 4%	8	—	8	—	—
CHG 2% with alcohol	12	—	13	—	—
Iodine	—	22	—	8	—
Iodine based with alcohol	2	—	—	14	—
PCMX	—	—	1	—	—
Sterile water	—	—	—	—	22

Results from an independent survey specific to this document. Information was obtained from surgical teams for a total of 22 surgeons in 9 hospitals.
Abbreviation: PCMX, parachlorometaxylenol.

The patient skin preparation protocol followed should be well documented in the patient data record.[15] Documentation should include assessment of the skin before the application of the antiseptic agent; location, time, and method of the preparation; name of the antiseptic agent applied; and the name of the practitioner who applied the skin preparation agent.

OFF-LABEL USE

To bring a product to market, the manufacturer conducts and supports research to determine product efficacy as well as product characteristics that are required by the FDA. All product label indications and directions for use are based on the results of multiple and varied clinical studies. If a practitioner or health care organization chooses to use a skin preparation product without complying with the manufacturer's written directions or labeled instructions, this use is considered off-label (eg, using an alcohol-based skin preparation product and not adhering to proper drying times). In addition, if a product is used off-label, the manufacturer cannot scientifically support the efficacy of the product because studies were not completed to support additional product claims.

Off-label use can become a challenge to perioperative nurses if they are either asked or instructed to use the product incorrectly.

WHAT IS THE IDEAL SKIN PREPARATION AGENT?

Postoperative infections occur in patients when the environment is supportive of bacterial growth. The selection of the surgical skin preparation agent should involve using good nursing assessment skills. Does the skin preparation agent show the following characteristics?

- Is there immediate and persistent action?
- Is it nontoxic and nonallergenic?
- Is it nonirritating?
- Does it have a broad spectrum of activity?
- Is it easy to use?
- What is the chance of flammability?
- What is the cost associated with it?

CONSIDERATIONS FOR PRACTICE

As discussed in this article, there are several skin preparation agents used in health care today. Based on the clinical impact of surgical-site infections, perioperative practitioners should consider the following key points[1,5,16]:

- The patient's skin should be free of any gross contamination, such as soil or other debris. At-home preoperative skin cleansing is the first order of the day before the surgical procedure, with a minimum of 2 skin cleansings using a 4% CHG product beginning at least the night before surgery
- The preoperative nurse should assess the patient to determine whether any allergies exist. The antiseptic agent should be selected based on the patient assessment
- Protective measures should be in place to preserve skin integrity and prevent injury to the skin such as pooling and other chemical burns
- Hand hygiene should be performed and sterile gloves donned by the perioperative practitioner performing the skin preparation before application

- If flammable agents such as tinctures are used, protective measures must be taken
- The skin preparation should be applied to the surgical site in concentric circles, beginning with the area of incision. The application should be wide enough to allow for extension of the incision or new incisions if they are necessary
- Perioperative practitioners should always follow manufacturer's instructions.

SUMMARY

Skin is the patient's first line of defense against infection. Because the skin cannot be sterilized, it must be properly prepared to reduce the microbial count to the lowest possible number, thereby reducing the risk of infection. Literature clearly shows that starting with clean skin and performing an appropriate skin antisepsis does protect the patient against bacteria before the incision. In their 1B Recommended Guideline, the CDC echoes these protocols[4]:

- Require patients to shower or bathe with an antiseptic agent on at least the night before the operative day.
- Thoroughly wash and clean at and around the incision site to remove gross contamination before performing antiseptic skin preparation.
- Use an appropriate antiseptic agent for skin preparation.

According to Dr R.L. Nichols, "The most critical factors in the prevention of postoperative infections, although difficult to quantify, are the sound judgment and proper technique of the surgeon and surgical team, as well as the general health and disease state of the patient."[2] There are 2 major opportunities for the reduction of skin flora associated with every patient's surgical journey. The first opportunity starts at home with the 4% CHG preoperative skin cleansing baths or showers, which affords the patient the opportunity to be a true partner in the fight against postoperative surgical infections.

The second opportunity begins with the preoperative surgical skin preparation. Careful patient assessment and appropriate application of antiseptic agents can make a difference. By using best-practice guidelines, perioperative practitioners can continue the fight to reduce postoperative infections.

REFERENCES

1. Mangran AJ, Horan TC, Pearson MI, et al. Guideline for prevention of surgical site infection, 1999. Hospital Infection Control Practices Advisory Committee. Infect Control Hosp Epidemiol 1999;20:250.
2. Nichols R. Preventing surgical site infections: a surgeon's perspective. Emerg Infect Dis 2001;7(2):220–4.
3. Lemmo, R. Combat surgical site infections before they enter your facility. Operating Room. p. 22–6. Available at: http://healthVIE.com 2010. Accessed January, 2011.
4. Appendix J. CDC Recommendation for the prevention of surgical site infections.1999. Adapted from Mangram, HICPAC and CDC. Available at: http://www.reproline.jhu.edu/english/4morerh/4ip/IP_manual/J_CDC%20Recommendations. Pdf. Accessed January, 2011.
5. AORN perioperative standards and recommended practices. RP Preoperative patient skin antisepsis. Denver (CO): the Association of Perioperative Registered Nurses. Copyright © 2009 AORN, Inc; 2010. p. 351–69.

6. Centers for Disease Control and Prevention. Guideline for hand hygiene in health-care settings. MMWR Recomm Rep 2002;51(RR-16):1–34.
7. Boyce JM, Pittet D. Guideline for hand hygiene in health-care settings. Recommendations of the Healthcare Infection Control Practice Advisory Committee and the HICPAC/SHEA/APIC/IDSA Hand hygiene Task Force. MMWR Recomm Rep 2002;51:1.
8. Darouiche R, Wall M, Itani K, et al. Chlorhexidine-alcohol versus povidone iodine for surgical-site antisepsis. N Engl J Med 2010;362(1):18–26.
9. Fletcher N, Sofianos D, Berkes M. Prevention of perioperative infection. J Bone Joint Surg Am 2007;89:1605–18.
10. Prasad R, Quezado Z, Andre A, et al. Fires in the operating room and intensive care unit: awareness is the key to prevention. Anesth Analg 2006;102:172–4.
11. Survey of standard operating room procedures. Sweet Haven Publishing Services. Available at: www.waybuilder.net/./Surgery02. Accessed December 3, 2010.
12. Rao N, Cannella B, Crossett L, et al. A preoperative decolonization protocol for *Staphylococcus aureus* prevents orthopaedic infections. Symposium: Papers Presented at the Fall 2007 Meeting of the Musculoskeletal Infection Society. Philadelphia, PA, June 2008. J Bone Surg Am 2008;466(6):1343–8. Available at: http://www.clinorthop.org/journal/11999/466/index.html.
13. Sorrentino S. Assisting with patient care. St Louis (MO): Mosby; 2006. p. 305–10.
14. Modified bed bath, skill 12. Harrisburg (PA): NNAAP; 2009.
15. Recommended standards of practice for skin prep of the surgical patient. Adapted from Core Curriculum for Surgical Assisting. 2nd edition. Littleton (CO): Association of Surgical Technologists; 2006.
16. Manring M, Calhoun J, Marculescu C. Minimizing the risk of post operative infection. Curr Orthop Pract 2009;20(4):429–36.

Special Considerations in History and Physical Assessment of the Plastic, Cosmetic, and Reconstructive Surgery Patient

Andrea Fassiotto, RN

KEYWORDS

- Patient history • Assessment • Plastic surgery
- Reconstructive surgery

One of the most important tasks of the perioperative nurse is to obtain a thorough history and physical assessment before surgery. This task is the first line of defense for safeguarding the surgical patients against potential complications. Many patients do not realize how their past medical and surgical history affects each future procedure, therefore it is critical to assess the patient for an accurate history. The nurse should be able to assess the patient, obtain a history of the patient, and observe for any potential problems.

The advent of electronic medical records (EMRs) has made this task much easier on nurses and patients alike. Patients who have been seen in your facility before will already have their records in the system. The history will just need to be reviewed and any updates made. For patients who have never visited your facility, it will make it easier to do a consistent interview, and their information will be in the system for any subsequent visits. However, not all facilities have EMRs at present, and paper files are still being kept. Whichever system your surgery center uses, remember to keep all records confidential in accordance with the HIPPA (US Health Insurance Portability and Accountability Act).

BUILDING PATIENT TRUST FOR OPTIMAL CARE

When obtaining a history and performing a physical examination, it is important to establish a rapport with the patient. Make sure she is comfortable, and provide for

Murray Calloway County Hospital, 803 Poplar Street, Murray, KY 42071, USA
E-mail address: afassiotto@murrayhospital.org

Perioperative Nursing Clinics 6 (2011) 125–129
doi:10.1016/j.cpen.2011.03.003
1556-7931/11/$ – see front matter © 2011 Elsevier Inc. All rights reserved.

periopnursing.theclinics.com

privacy. Minimize distractions, and make eye contact with your patients to reassure them that you are listening to what they say.

Does the patient have any religious or cultural beliefs that would affect her care? Some cultures are more private than others or regard eye contact as being rude. In addition, members of the Jehovah's Witness religion do not accept any blood products. Most facilities will require patients to sign a release of responsibility if they need a transfusion but refuse it.

Most of us have a routine when we are obtaining a history and performing a physical assessment. We also make many system observations at once when we initially meet our patient. How many times have you noticed patients' pain, nausea, or nervousness as soon as they walked in?

CREATE A CONSISTENT, SYSTEMATIC APPROACH

A systematic approach to doing the history and physical assessment works best. Take each body system individually, asking patients questions regarding each system. Some nurses do their assessment and history together, others ask questions first and then move on to the assessment. Whichever technique you use, consistency is the key. When you use the same technique with each patient, you are less likely to overlook the key points of your assessment.

The integumentary system is a good place to start. Patients' skin can tell us a great deal about their overall well-being. Does she have any rash, cut, or bruis or any skin condition such as psoriasis? Has she ever had a wound that would not heal, an infection caused by methicillin-resistant *Staphylococcus aureus*, or a vancomycin-resistant infection? Ask the patient to show you any unusual skin conditions.

Has she had any history of any neurologic disorder? Ask the patient about headaches, including migraines. Does she have any history of seizures? If so, are they well controlled? When was the last one? Are the seizures petit or grand mal? Is the patient alert and oriented to person, place, and time? Does she have any slurred speech? Does the patient answer questions in a timely manner?

The patient's cardiac history should include asking about high or low blood pressure. Does she have high cholesterol or a history of irregular heartbeats or mitral valve prolapse? Does she have any congenital heart abnormalities? Auscultation of heart sounds should reveal no abnormalities. There should be no peripheral edema or jugular venous distension. Blood pressure and pulse should be within the normal limits.

ASSESSING THE BODY SYSTEMS

The respiratory system should reveal a patient who breathes without difficulty and has no signs of cyanosis. Lung sounds should be clear anteriorly and posteriorly. The sounds should also be clear on inspiration and expiration. Does she have any history of asthma or chronic obstructive pulmonary disease? Does she smoke? If so, how many packs per day and for how many years? Offer the patient counseling to help her quit.

Ask the patient if she has any sleep apnea and if she uses continuous pulmonary airway pressure or bilevel positive airway pressure at night when sleeping.

The gastrointestinal system assessment should include questions regarding difficulty swallowing, heartburn, and stomach discomfort; recent unintended weight loss or gain; and bowel habits. Does she have any dietary concerns or restrictions? We are beginning to see many patients who have had surgeries to help with obesity. Those patients will have various restrictions based on their doctor's preference. Ask her about any history of gastroesophageal reflux disease, irritable bowel syndrome, Crohn disease, or ulcerative colitis. The abdomen should be soft and nontender without masses. The nurse should be able to auscultate bowel sounds in all 4 quadrants.

This may be a good opportunity to discuss weight management with patients who are having a cosmetic procedure to remove excess skin. How much weight have they lost? Do they have a reasonable plan in place to maintain that weight loss? Are they participating in an exercise program? A nutritional consult may be warranted at this time.

Assessment of the genitourinary system includes asking the patient about any difficulty with urination, kidney stones, excessive or diminished urination, stress incontinence, or pain. Urine should be clear yellow, without blood or odor. Physical assessment of this system can be deferred to the physician if a problem has been found.

The reproductive system will have more questions that are gender specific to women. The nurse will need to ask about her last menstrual period. Has she had any children? And if so, how many? Does she plan on any more children? Did she breastfeed? When was her last Papanicolaou test? Does the patient do regular breast/testicular examinations? Is there any history of sexually transmitted diseases? Does the patient have any lump in the breasts or any nipple discharge? Men can have those too, so they should not be left out.

The endocrine system can reveal possible comorbidities, such as diabetes and hypothyroidism. If the patient is diabetic, is it well controlled? Does the patient have excessive thirst or urination and any recent hair loss?

The eye, ear, nose, and throat can be assessed together. The patient should have no complaints of hearing or vision changes. Nose and throat should be clear. Ask the patient about any seasonal allergies. The trachea should be midline. Patient should not have any difficulty swallowing. No swollen lymph nodes should be noted to the neck. Patient should not have any difficulty moving his head or neck.

The nurse begins to assess the musculoskeletal system as soon as the patient walks on to the unit. It is subconsciously done by watching patients as they move. Do they have any difficulty with walking? Do they have any visible abnormalities, such as a limp or an amputation? Has the patient had any past traumas, muscle pains, or strains? Is the patient able to do the activities of daily living? Knowing this information may help determine if the patient will be able to care for herself according to her doctor's advice after she goes home.

THE WHOLE PICTURE

The patient's surgical history is important, because it helps understand how well they did with past procedures. Did the patient have postoperative nausea and vomiting? Did the patient experience difficulty waking up? Did the patient have to be placed on a ventilator? Does the patient or any of his or her family have a history of malignant hyperthermia? Answers to these questions could give the anesthesia provider clues to any possible problems with anesthesia.

A patient also brings her family history to the table anytime she has a procedure. Family history can play an important role because of the potential problems it can cause for the patient. Does her family have a strong history of heart disease or cancer? Is there a history of any familial bleeding disorder such as hemophilia or von Willebrand disease? Does she have a significant occurrence of diabetes in her family? Ask the patient to limit the family history to the immediate family only.

Patients often take several medications a day. Knowing what those medicines are can clue a nurse in to what is going on with the patient and help avert potential problems with any medications she may receive during her surgery. Ask the patient to include all medications including over-the-counter medicines. Also have the patient include herbal and vitamin supplements. Many patients do not realize that supplements can also affect them adversely with other medications. What dosage is each medicine, and how many times a day does the patient take her medicine?

Drug, environmental, and food allergies should also be assessed. A patient with a latex allergy should ideally be the first case of the day in that surgical suite. Many drugs are related to each other, so it is important to know what drugs the patient is allergic to and what kind of reaction the drug caused. Food allergies are also key because several medications have a food base, such as eggs. We would want to avoid all egg-based products for this patient.

Laboratory values vary from physician to physician and facility to facility. The nurse will want to check to see if the patient has had her laboratory work completed. She will also want to evaluate the laboratory work for any abnormalities that need to be alerted to the physician before surgery.

PATIENT-SPECIFIC AND PROCEDURE-SPECIFIC ASSESSMENT

Questions and assessments may be specific to each procedure. A patient undergoing rhinoplasty will have a different approach from a patient undergoing abdominoplasty or breast reduction. A patient having rhinoplasty will need to have more questions directed toward respiratory and facial concerns. The patient undergoing abdominoplasty will need questions regarding the abdomen and weight loss and gain. What about the possibility of children after surgery? A woman who will be having breast reduction will have more questions regarding back, shoulder, and neck pain. It is imperative to individualize each assessment for each patient and procedure.

Many cosmetic procedures have a photography session. This is to take a photograph of the before-surgery assessment. This is usually an awkward time for the patient. The procedure she is having done may be because of a body flaw that has caused her a great deal of embarrassment over the years. Try to put your patient at ease by providing privacy and explaining that this will be kept confidential. Many facilities have computer-generated images of what the patient will look like after the procedure. Follow your facility's protocol in going over these images with your patient. Let your patient know how any photography may be used, and make sure you have obtained the right to use those photographs.

What are the patient's expectations of the surgery? Are they realistic? Some patients have grandiose ideas of what cosmetic surgery can do to their lives, and it is crucial to find out what the patient expects to happen after surgery. What kind of coping mechanisms does she have in place? Does she have supportive people around her? This could be important to know when discussing patient satisfaction with her procedure postoperatively.

Obtaining a thorough history and physical assessment is a critical step for nurses to undertake in keeping the patients safe during surgery. Each physician and facility has its own routine, but all share the common goal of providing the highest quality of care possible to every patient, and during every surgery. A complete assessment, attention to detail, and patient education may help ensure better outcomes as well as avoid potential complications.

FURTHER READINGS

Assessment made incredibly easy. In: Jackson K, Hendler B, Tscheschlog BA, editors. 2nd edition. Springhouse (PA);2002. p. 3–318.

Mosby's expert physical exam handbook: rapid inpatient and outpatient assessments. St Louis (MO): Mosby; 2009. All Chapters.

Odom-Forren J, Watson D. Practical guide to moderate sedation/analgesia. 2nd edition. Presadation assessment, monitoring parameters, and equipment. St Louis (MO): Elsevier Mosby; 2005. p. 20–52. Chapter 2.

Seidel HM, Ball WJ, Dains JE, et al. Mosby's Guide to Physical Examination. St Louis (MO): Mosby Elsevier; 2010. Chapters 1, 2, and 3.

Spector D, Mayer DK, Knafl K, et al. Not what I expected informational needs of women undergoing breast surgery. Plastic Surgical Nursing 2010;30(2):70–4.

Surgical care made incredibly visual preoperative care. In: Buss JS, editor. Springhouse (PA): Lippincott Williams & Wilkins; 2006.

Laser-Assisted Liposuction

Alberto Goldman, MD[a],*, Robert H. Gotkin, MD[b]

KEYWORDS

• Laser lipolysis • Laser-assisted liposuction • Nd YAG laser

Over the past 30 years, liposuction has become an increasingly popular procedure. According to the American Society for Aesthetic Plastic Surgery, liposuction has been the most commonly performed cosmetic surgical procedure every year of this decade.[1] From its modern reinvention over 30 years ago, in which large uterine curettes and gynecologic aspirators were used to remove fat,[2,3] to the myriad technological advances that exist today, liposuction has undergone many changes. These changes can be divided into three main categories: changes in anesthesia management, changes in equipment and cannula size, and changes in the actual methods of treating and removing fat.

In the 1980s, liposuction usually was performed as a hospital inpatient procedure under general anesthesia, and it often required transfusion of autologous blood to replace that which was lost during the procedure. In 1988, Klein[4] published his landmark article on the tumescent technique; this method of administering large quantities of very dilute buffered lidocaine and epinephrine significantly reduced intraoperative blood loss and allowed the procedure to be moved from an inpatient setting to an office or other outpatient setting. Although slow to be adopted by many plastic surgeons, when properly used, Klein's tumescent technique dramatically improved the safety of liposuction and became incorporated into the procedure.[5]

The dramatic reduction in intraoperative blood loss and postoperative ecchymoses improved the recovery for patients undergoing liposuction. Surgeons continued to refine the procedure with the addition of internal ultrasound-assisted liposuction,[6–8] external ultrasound-assisted lipoplasty,[9] and power-assisted lipoplasty.[10] Parallel to these developments, Apfelberg[11–13] was beginning to study laser-assisted liposuction; this preliminary investigation utilized a YAG optical fiber contained within a liposuction cannula. The investigators concluded that no clear benefit was demonstrated with the laser; the US Food and Drug Administration (FDA) did not approve the

A version of this article was previously published in the *Clinics in Plastic Surgery* 36:2.

The authors have no significant financial interest in any of the companies mentioned herein.

[a] Clinica Goldman of Plastic Surgery, Avenue Augusto Meyer 163 Conj. 1203, Porto Alegre, RS, Brazil 90550-110

[b] Cosmetique Dermatology, Laser & Plastic Surgery, LLP, 625 Park Avenue, New York, NY 10065, USA

* Corresponding author.

E-mail address: alberto@goldman.com.br

Perioperative Nursing Clinics 6 (2011) 131–145

doi:10.1016/j.cpen.2011.03.004

1556-7931/11/$ – see front matter © 2011 Elsevier Inc. All rights reserved.

technique, and the sponsoring laser company did not pursue the study. In the late 1990s, Neira and colleagues began studying the effects of low-level laser on adipose tissue.[14–17] At the same time, Blugerman[18] and Blugerman, Schavelzon, and Goldman[19–21] were using 1064 nm neodymium:yttrium-aluminum-garnet (Nd:YAG) laser energy, conducted by means of an optical fiber, within a 1 mm introducer cannula, in direct contact with adipose tissue. They found that the energy from the laser resulted in adipocyte lysis and other salutary side effects of the procedure and patient recovery. Badin and colleagues[22,23] arrived at very similar findings: less intra-operative blood loss, less postoperative ecchymoses, and improved skin tightening and skin redraping during the recovery process.

These findings have spurred a tremendous interest in laser lipolysis and laser-assisted liposuction. With the broad approval by the FDA in October 2006, of a 1064 nm Nd:YAG laser (Smartlipo, Cynosure, Incorporated, Westford, MA, USA) for surgical incision, excision, vaporization, ablation and coagulation in soft tissues, and laser lipolysis, this interest has become even more magnified. Other lasers also have received FDA approval in the United States, and it appears that laser-assisted liposuction, although just one of many tools in the armamentarium of the aesthetic surgeon performing body contouring, has emerged as a hot technique in aesthetic plastic surgery.

SCIENCE

The laser–tissue interaction in adipose tissue has been described by many investigators.[11–28] Whether the laser acts directly upon the fat[18–25] or whether it is administered transcutaneously,[14–17] the final common pathway appears to be similar. Neira,[14–17] Goldman,[24] Ichikawa,[25] and their respective colleagues have elucidated this.

Neira's technique involved the external, transcutaneous application of low-level laser energy using a 635 nm diode laser with a maximum power of 10 mW. Even at these low energy delivery levels, Neira found a time- and, therefore, dose-dependent effect of laser energy on adipocytes. This was contrasted with a control population that received only tumescent solution without exposure to laser energy. At exposure times of 4 minutes, there was partial disruption of about 80% of the adipo-cytes' cell membranes. At longer exposure times (6 minutes), there was almost complete disruption in 99% of adipocyte cell membranes. In addition to this lipolysis, the laser energy also appeared to disrupt adipose connective tissue. In the control group, there was no change in the size, shape, or integrity of the adipocytes. With the spillage of intracellular contents into the extracellular or interstitial space, there was easier fat extraction, a reduction in surgical trauma, and a more abbreviated post-operative recovery.

Although these findings could not be confirmed independently by Brown and colleagues,[26] Ichikawa and colleagues[25] subsequently showed the histologic findings in fat subjected to direct treatment with the 1064 nm Nd:YAG laser. In both photomi-croscopic and scanning electron microscopic studies, Ichikawa demonstrated greater destruction of human adipocytes in laser-irradiated fat compared with nonlaser-irradiated controls. There seemed to be a dose-dependent degeneration of adipocyte cell membranes, vaporization and liquefaction of fat cells, and collagen fiber coagula-tion in response to the 1064 nm Nd:YAG laser irradiation.

With an Nd:YAG laser in direct contact with adipose tissue, Goldman[20,24] and Badin[22,23] demonstrated adipocyte cell membrane rupture, coagulation of small vessels within the adipose tissue, coagulation of adipose and dermal collagen, and a reorganization of the reticular dermis (**Figs. 1** and **2**). The latter is associated with a process of neocollagenesis in the deep dermis and the dermal fat junction. These histologic findings seem to correlate with the clinical findings of a reduction in intraoperative blood loss, reduction in postoperative ecchymoses, a more comfortable postoperative recovery, a rapid return to activities of daily living (ADL), and enhanced skin tightening and skin redraping as a result of the neocollagenesis.

Kim and Geronemus[27] also confirmed similar findings; the lipolysis produced by the Nd:YAG laser acting in adipose tissue is an elegant and minimally invasive option associated with demonstrable reduction in fat volume, irrespective of subject weight change. There was excellent patient tolerance and the benefit of dermal tightening. The postoperative recovery was quick, and patients had a rapid return to ADL. MRI studies performed before and 3 months following surgery showed an average 17% reduction in adipose tissue volume in the areas treated; site-specific analysis revealed a 25% reduction in the submental area and an overall 14% reduction in the trunk and extremities.

Mordon and colleagues,[28] also demonstrated similar clinical and histologic findings using a continuous-wave 980 nm diode laser (Pharaon [Osyris; Hellemmes, France] and Lipotherme [MedSurge Advances, Dallas, TX, USA]). At similar power settings as the pulsed Nd:YAG, the histologic findings were similar. This laser has the capability of higher wattage than the Nd:YAG laser; however, at these higher powers, there was carbonization noted in the adipose tissue and collagen fibers. This is significant, because carbonization and charring of tissues is much more likely to lead to unfavorable and unacceptable scarring internally and possibly externally. Perhaps the different pulse profile may be responsible for this; the continuous-wave diode and the pulsed Nd:YAG interact with adipose tissue in a different manner. The continuous waveform is more likely to char the tissues than a high peak power, but short duration pulsed waveform. The latter is more in harmony with the thermal relaxation time of the tissues.

The mechanism of action on a cellular level is caused by a specific laser–tissue interaction that is defined by the process of selective photothermolysis[29]; some features of this interaction are wavelength-dependent, and some are independent of wavelength used. There are three wavelengths currently on the market in the United States for laser lipolysis: pulsed 1064 nm, pulsed 1320 nm, and CW 980 nm diode. All three wavelengths generate infrared light energy that is absorbed by adipocytes and converted to heat. This absorption of energy causes deformation of the adipocyte, volume expansion and, subsequently, cell rupture. The adipocytes exposed to the highest energies undergo a photoacoustic or photomechanical disruption; those exposed to

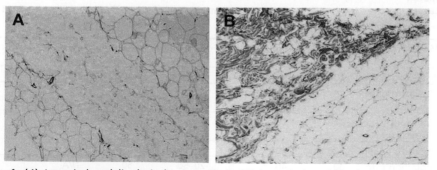

Fig. 1. (*A*) Laser-induced lipolysis (H & E: 40×). (*B*) Laser-induced lipolysis and adipose collagen coagulation (H & E: 40×).

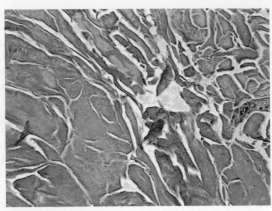

Fig. 2. Collagen coagulation (H & E: 100×).

lower energies (further from the tip of the optical fiber) undergo a photothermal change. The latter results in cellular deformation and expansion, but may not lead to immediate rupture; because of the changes in membrane permeability, however, many of these cells eventually die. The cellular debris is metabolized, and the metabolic by-products are excreted by means of the liver or kidneys. An additional effect of the laser-induced heating of the tissues appears to be a photostimulatory effect; this phenomenon is a lower energy process that occurs even further from the fiber tip and has broad overall activity on dermal and adipose collagen.

The 1064 nm wavelength also is known to be absorbed by oxyhemoglobin, and has even better absorption by methemoglobin (**Fig. 2**). Because of these absorption characteristics, this wavelength is effective in coagulating small blood vessels within the fat and seems to be responsible for the histologic and clinical findings noted by several investigators.[18–25]

As of June 2008, there were four devices approved by the FDA for laser lipolysis in the United States (**Table 1**). The pulsed 1064 nm Nd:YAG laser (Smartlipo [Cynosure; DEKA, Calenzano, Italy]) used for laser lipolysis has a pulse width of 100 milliseconds; the default energy delivery is 150 mJ/pulse and 40 Hz, but the energy per pulse and the

Table 1
Lasers approved by the US Food and Drug Administration for laser lipolysis as of June 2008

	Smartlipo	Smartlipo-MPX	CoolLipo	LipoLite	Lipotherme
Manufacturer	Cynosure	Cynosure	CoolTouch	Syneron	Osyris/Med Surge Advances
Wavelength (nm)	1064	1064, 1320	1320	1064	980 diode
Maximum power (watts)	18	20, 12	15	?	25
Pulse width (μsec)	100	150	100	100–800	(CW)
Fiber size (s) (μm)	300, 600	600	200, 320, 500	550	600
Repetition rate	40	40	20–50	50	N/A
Pulse energy (mJ)	150	500, 300	?	<250–800	N/A

pulses per second settings are variable. The original laser marketed in the United States and internationally had a maximum power of 6 W; this has been increased to 18 W as a stand-alone 1064 nm Nd:YAG laser. Cynosure now also markets a 1064 nm and 1320 nm multiplexed system with a maximum of 20 watts at 1064 nm and 12 W at 1320 nm. The 1064 nm pulse width is 150 milliseconds, and the 1320 nm pulse width is 212 milliseconds. Either wavelength can be used alone, or the two can be used together in a multiplexed fashion. The original 6 W laser came with an optical fiber of 300 μm in diameter; a 600 μm diameter fiber is also available. Both can be passed through a 1 mm microcannula; however the 600 μm fiber passes more easily through a 1.5 mm external diameter microcannula. The larger fiber and the larger microcannula, and the higher-powered lasers, are more robust and efficient for lipolysis.

The different absorption characteristics of the 1064 nm and 1320 nm wavelengths are responsible for their distinctive actions in adipose tissue. As noted in **Fig. 3**, the 1320 nm wavelength has a higher coefficient of absorption in water than the 1064 nm wavelength. In adipose tissue, this wavelength is strongly absorbed with less scattering compared with the 1064 nm wavelength. Therefore, the 1320 nm wavelength is extremely effective at rapidly heating adipose tissue in a very localized manner; most of the energy is absorbed in a small region immediately around the tip of the optical fiber. This is in contrast to the 1064 nm wavelength, in which energy diffuses over a broader treatment area, with a more controlled temperature elevation, more generalized heating of the fat, and better activity in hemoglobin. With water as the target chromophore of the 1320 nm wavelength, there is also a much greater effect on dermal collagen; this results in improved collagen shrinkage and skin tightening.

CoolTouch (Roseville, CA, USA) markets a 1320 nm Nd:YAG laser for laser lipolysis (CoolLipo). This pulsed Nd:YAG also has a pulse width of 100 milliseconds, power up to 15 W and a repetition of 20 to 50 Hz. Available optical fibers are 200, 320, and 500 μm in diameter. This device received FDA approval for laser-assisted lipolysis in January 2008.

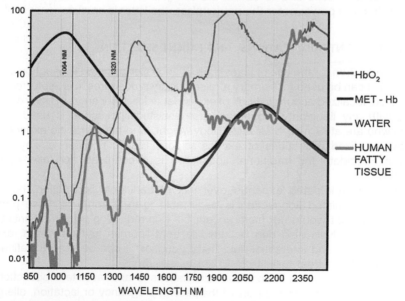

Fig. 3. Coefficients of absorption of water and human fatty tissue.

Syneron (Yokneam, Israel) received FDA clearance for laser lipolysis for its entry into the laser-assisted liposuction market (LipoLite) in May 2008. This laser is also a pulsed 1064 nm Nd:YAG, but features a variable pulse width (100 to 800 milliseconds) and variable pulse energy (<250 to 800 mJ per pulse). It fires up to 50 Hz, but the power is not specified.

The other device currently available in the United States for direct internal interaction with adipose tissue is the 980 nm diode laser (Lipotherme [MedSurge Advances, Dallas, TX, USA]).[28] Other companies have similar devices in their pipelines, but are awaiting FDA clearance. Because the 1064 nm Nd:YAG laser has been available in the United States and FDA-approved for the longest period of time compared with the other devices, it is the most studied regarding its clinical and histological effects and has the most prior publications.

Studies on the thermal energy generated in laser lipolysis are beginning to reveal important information on correlations between skin surface temperature and skin shrinkage or contraction. Patients undergoing laser lipolysis had tattoos placed to mark the abdominal and thigh skin in 5 cm square areas. The laser lipolysis was conducted with a multiplexed device emitting 1064 nm energy at 20 watts and 1320 nm energy at 12 watts. The procedure was performed in order to obtain the usual clinical endpoints for aesthetically pleasing body contouring. The square areas were measured at 3 months and revealed an average 18% contraction (Barry DiBernardo, MD and Bruce Katz, MD, personal communication, June, 2008). In the authors' opinion, this contraction is likely to increase somewhat over the next 3 months, as the clinical end point in the healing process has not been reached.

In addition, the optimal skin surface temperature necessary in order to obtain maximal skin contraction, without carbonization or excessive thermal injury, is being studied. It appears that this optimum temperature is between 35° and 40°C. With the tip of the optical fiber 5 mm below the skin surface, the maximum skin surface temperature before tissue necrosis noted is 47°C (Bruce Katz, MD, personal communication, 2008). These types of data are very important in order to obtain the best possible clinical results and to define the safety limits of the procedure. As more devices with more power enter the marketplace, the latter is crucial.

INDICATIONS, CONTRAINDICATIONS, AND PATIENT SELECTION

The main indication for the use of laser lipolysis and laser-assisted liposuction is body contouring. It can be used for primary and secondary procedures; it is useful for small, well-defined, localized accumulations of excess fat or for larger areas of body contouring. As with any lipoplasty technique, laser-assisted liposuction is used best in patients who are at or near their ideal body weight, who have realistic expectations and have localized collections of excess adipose tissue. In essence, any patient who is a candidate for traditional liposuction is a candidate for laser-assisted liposuction.

The field of candidates expands over that of traditional liposuction, however, because laser-assisted liposuction is better able to treat some of those patients with skin laxity that would not have acceptable skin redraping with traditional techniques. Laser lipolysis also can be used to treat lipomas, gynecomastia, axillary hyperhidrosis,[30,31] and interstitial fluid malar pouches; it can be used to refine and contour flaps and to treat cellulite.[32]

Similar to traditional liposuction, contraindications to laser-assisted liposuction are unrealistic expectations on the part of the patient, pregnancy or lactation, allergy to lidocaine, and any general medical issues that would prevent someone from being able to have local anesthesia. If the procedure is to be performed under intravenous sedation, epidural block or general anesthesia (usually because of being combined with other procedures) the patient must be in good general medical condition to undergo such anesthetic management. The authors have found no procedure-specific contraindications to laser-assisted liposuction.

In selecting appropriate patients for this procedure, the surgeon should apply many of the dictums that apply to traditional liposuction. The preoperative consultation should include an evaluation of the patient's goals and expectations. If the procedure is being performed for purposes of body contouring, the areas of accumulation of excess fat should be delineated; the quality, thickness, turgor, and elasticity of the overlying skin should be determined. The pinch test, an important maneuver for any experienced liposuction surgeon, should be employed preoperatively to evaluate skin thickness, skin elasticity, and adipose thickness; intraoperatively to monitor the progress of the procedure; and postoperatively to evaluate the quality of the result.

If the laser is being utilized to treat axillary hyperhidrosis, it is helpful to employ a starch–iodine test preoperatively in order to precisely define the areas of greatest sweat production. This should be performed, photographed, measured, and compared with the postoperative result. When laser lipolysis is used to treat gyneco-mastia or to thin or contour a flap, there is essentially no difference in the preoperative evaluation or patient selection compared with traditional liposuction.

If laser lipolysis is being employed to treat cellulite, not only are the areas of cellulite important to evaluate preoperatively, but other areas that may benefit from body con-touring need to be examined also. The importance here lies in the potential donor sites for autologous fat transplantation; this donor fat must be harvested with traditional liposuction—not with laser-assisted liposuction—so as to maintain the integrity and viability of the adipocytes for transplantation.[32,33] Autologous fat is very useful to enhance the deepest, most concave areas of contour deformity in the correction of cellulite.

TECHNIQUE

Laser-assisted liposuction may be performed under local anesthesia alone, or supple-mented with intravenous sedation, epidural block, or general anesthesia. This is an individual choice between the surgeon and the patient. Irrespective of anesthetic choice, the patient is marked in the standing position. If treatment is for cellulite, it is helpful to use various markers of different colors in order to mark areas of elevation and depression.[32] Once marked, the patient is brought to the operating room and prepped circumferentially in the standing position.[33] Following the preparation, the patient is placed on the operating table upon sterile drapes; this will allow the patient to be turned during the procedure without having to re-prep.[34,35] A single intravenous dose of a first- generation cephalosporin usually is administered.

If the procedure is expected to last 1 hour or more, external pneumatic compression devices (eg, Venodyne, Columbus, MI, USA) are placed on the legs, and the patient is sedated if desired. Subcutaneous infiltration of warmed Klein's tumescent solution, or some similar solution combining buffered lidocaine and epinephrine, precedes laser application to the areas of unwanted fat. Klein's solution contains 500 mg lidocaine, 1 mg epinephrine and 12.5 cc of 8.4% $NaHCO_3$ per liter of normal saline. This makes a buffered solution containing approximately 0.05% lidocaine, 1:1,000,000 units epinephrine. The total volume of subcutaneous infiltration depends upon surgeon preference and the overall size of the treatment area. The solution is warmed to mini-mize any discomfort associated with a temperature difference between the tissue and

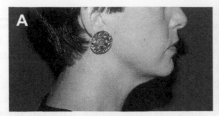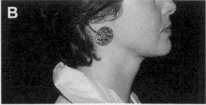

Fig. 4. 44-year-old woman is shown before (*A*) and 6 months after (*B*) laser-assisted liposuction of the neck.

the fluid. Warming also helps to maintain core body temperature. The procedure is initiated following a 10- to 20-minute delay to allow for appropriate diffusion of the fluid and adequate vasoconstriction. Neira[15] compared longer laser energy exposure times in the absence of tumescent solution with shorter exposure times in the presence of tumescent solution. His histologic findings were comparable in the two groups, and he concluded that the tumescent solution enhanced the laser's activity on adipocytes.

Direct laser application into the adipose tissue occurs by means of an optical fiber. This fiber (200 to 600 μm in diameter) is conducted within a stainless steel microcannula of 1 to 1.5 mm external diameter. An important distinction between the current laser-assisted liposuction and that investigated by Apfelberg[11–13] in the 1990s is the location of the tip of the optical fiber. In Apfelberg's study, the tip of the fiber was within the liposuction cannula so that only that fat that had been avulsed already by the suction was exposed to the activity of the laser. All current systems work by having the tip of the fiber extend beyond the end of the cannula by 2 to 3 mm. This 2 to 3 mm extension enables the direct activity of laser energy within the adipose tissue. The optical fiber is conducted by means of very fine, small-diameter instruments, and no high negative pressure suction occurs. Lipolysis and small vessel and collagen coagulation occur directly by means of the activity of the laser. This distinction has further importance relative to the minimally invasive nature of the procedure.

The optical fiber conducts both the therapeutic infrared light (980, 1064, or 1320 nm) and a helium–neon aiming beam (634 nm). The transillumination of the HeNe beam allows for precise localization of the fiber tip so that the surgeon is constantly aware of the location of laser activity. The intensity of the aiming beam is also clinically relevant. The brighter the intensity of the beam, the more superficial within the tissue the fiber tip is located. Conversely, a lower intensity transillumination of the HeNe beam means that the tip of the fiber is deeper in the tissues.

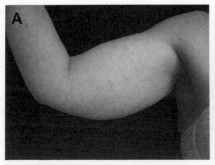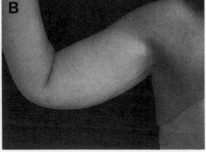

Fig. 5. 54-year-old woman is shown before (*A*) and 8 months after (*B*) laser-assisted liposuction of the arms.

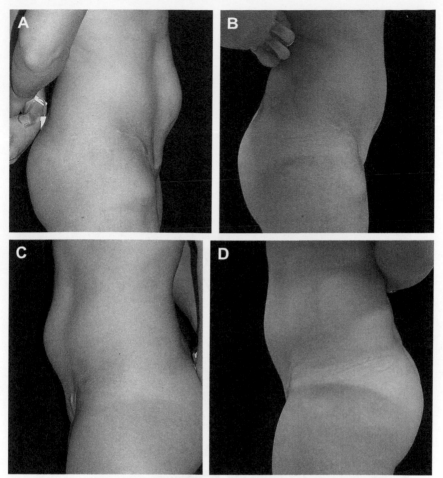

Fig. 6. 26-year-old woman is shown before (*A, C*) and 6 months after (*B, D*) laser-assisted liposuction of the abdomen.

Other delivery systems are beginning to enter the marketplace. The two most significant new delivery systems are a combination laser application–suction cannula (CoolTouch) and a motion-sensing feedback hand piece (Cynosure). The former combines simultaneous aspiration with laser application by enclosing the fiber in a small-diameter suction cannula; this cannula has a Y shape at the proximal end to accommodate the entry of the fiber and the connection for aspiration tubing. Other manufacturers are developing similar delivery systems.

Cynosure's SmartSense hand piece contains a motion-sensing feedback chip that feeds back information on the movement of the cannula to the laser device; this enables the laser to shut down energy delivery if it senses cessation of cannula movement. This safety feature helps to prevent overaccumulation of thermal energy in a given area and, therefore, helps to prevent carbonization, burns, and consequent adverse scarring.

The duration of laser activity in the tissues is highly variable and depends upon the overall size of the treatment area, the thickness and volume of fat being removed, the degree of skin laxity, and the presence of previous internal scarring (eg, a secondary

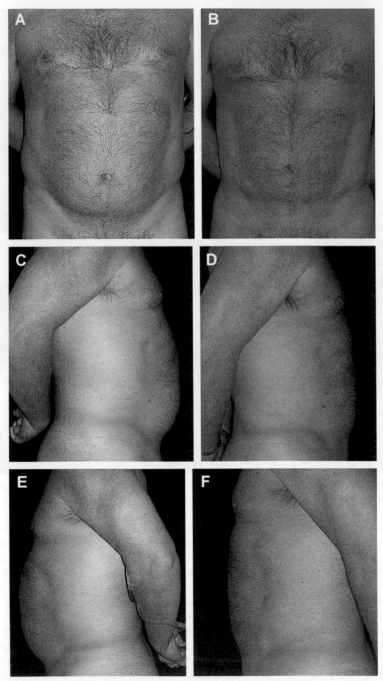

Fig. 7. 47-year-old man before (*A, C, E, G*) and 6 months after (*B, D, F, H*) laser-assisted liposuction of the abdomen, hips, and flanks.

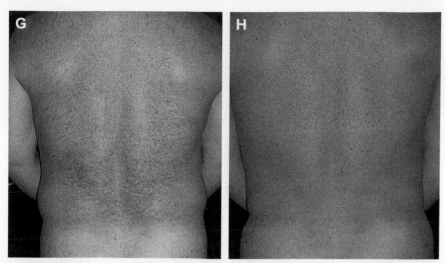

Fig. 7. (*continued*)

procedure). The surgeon senses a diminishing resistance to cannula movement as the procedure progresses. This indicates lipolysis and the presence of more liquefied fat (lysate) and less normal, untreated fat. As mentioned previously, the pinch test is another important factor in determining the clinical end point of treatment.

The resultant product of laser-assisted lipolysis is an oily lysate containing ruptured adipocytes and cellular debris mixed with tumescent solution. Aspiration of this lysate is the surgeon's choice. If the surgeon chooses to remove the mixture, it is removed by gentle aspiration using a 2 mm or 3 mm external diameter cannula and a negative pressure of 0.3 to 0.5 atm (<50 kPa or 350 mm Hg). In this way, the minimally invasive nature of the procedure is preserved; high negative pressure suction that is traumatic to the tissues is avoided, and the postoperative recovery period is enhanced. It is the authors' experience that very small areas of treatment with low volumes of lysate do well without aspiration. This may be the case, for example, in the treatment of the anterior cervical area. In situations when minimal lipolysis is desired, and the laser is being used mainly for the photostimulatory effect of collagen contraction, here, too, it may not be necessary to aspirate. This latter example often applies to the treatment of cellulite.

Hemoglobin, hematocrit, serum cholesterol, and serum triglycerides were measured in 20 patients in the preoperative period and 1 day, 1 week and 1 month following laser-assisted liposuction. No significant changes were noted.[20]

Following surgery, the use of compression garments is, again, the individual surgeon's choice. As long as they are not too constrictive, the garments are usually helpful in reducing edema and improving skin redraping. During the first 1 to 2 weeks following the procedure, the patient may be started on a postoperative physiotherapeutic routine to hasten the resolution of edema. Devices such as the Tri-Active (Cynosure), Endermologie (LPG; Cedex, France), VelaShape or VelaSmooth (Syneron) may be employed.

RESULTS

Laser lipolysis and laser-assisted liposuction have proven to be safe and effective methods of body contouring. Although the early clinical results may be similar to those

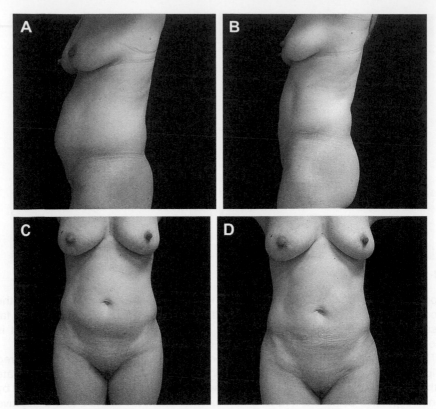

Fig. 8. 38-year-old woman is shown before (*A, C*) and 6 months after (*B, D*) laser-assisted liposuction of the abdomen, hips, and flanks.

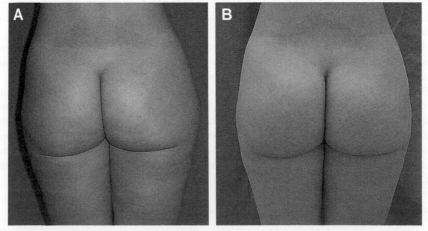

Fig. 9. 32-year-old woman is shown before (*A*) and 6 months after (*B*) laser-assisted liposuction of hips and thighs for treatment of cellulite.

obtained by traditional liposuction, the histologic findings suggest explanations for the differences being seen in the clinical course of recovery and the final clinical result. The coagulation of blood vessels noted histologically correlates with the reduction in perioperative and postoperative bleeding and ecchymoses. The coagulation of collagen in the adipose tissue and the deep dermis, associated with neocollagenesis and reorganization of the reticular dermis, explains the skin contraction or shrinkage noted in the later postoperative course. This capacity of the laser to produce skin contraction is very important in the treatment of patients with some degree of skin laxity who may not be candidates for traditional liposuction (**Figs. 4–10**).

Like traditional liposuction, laser-assisted liposuction is useful in combination with other surgical procedures such as facelift, abdominoplasty, thighplasty, reduction mammaplasty, and breast reconstruction. In the absence of platysmal banding, when used in the neck, laser-assisted liposuction may preclude having to open the neck in a facelift. In the surgical body-contouring procedures, it is helpful to contour the peripheral or adjacent areas not directly affected by dermatolipectomy.

COMPLICATIONS

Side effects and complications of laser-assisted liposuction are rare, and most do not appear to be specific for the use of the laser. The exception is thermal injury. The energy produced at the fiber tip can build up to harmful and damaging levels rather promptly if the surgeon's attention is diverted. Excessive subcutaneous or cutaneous thermal injury can occur. Any other potential complication or side effect noted with traditional liposuction can occur with laser-assisted liposuction also. There will be minimal ecchymoses, some edema, and the usual cutaneous anesthesia noted following traditional liposuction. When laser treatment is very superficial—in order to obtain maximal skin contraction or in the treatment of cellulite—the cutaneous

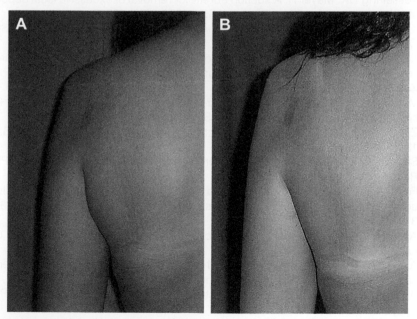

Fig. 10. 28-year-old woman is shown before (A) and 6 months after (B) laser-assisted liposuction of the posterior axillary area.

anesthesia may last somewhat longer.[32] Similar to traditional liposuction, minor aesthetic differences or asymmetries are the most common complication. As more powerful devices populate the market, greater care will have to be exercised to avoid thermal injuries.

SUMMARY

The ongoing search for new tools and alternative techniques in liposuction is related to an underlying desire of surgeons to improve the safety of the technique, reduce the downtime for patients, and enhance the ultimate cosmetic result. By reducing blood loss, minimizing both aesthetic and anesthetic side effects and complications, and by promoting improvements in skin contraction and redraping following surgery, laser-assisted liposuction has proven itself to be a safe, effective, and useful addition to the armamentarium of the plastic surgeon performing body contouring. A growing body of experience and evidence indicates that the technique can expand the base of patients who are candidates for primary liposuction as well as those who desire secondary procedures. The fact that this small-caliber, minimally invasive technology can be utilized very superficially, without leaving a footprint in the tissue, while coagulating collagen, inducing neocollagenesis and the accompanying skin contraction, is a tremendous advantage to surgeon and patient.

REFERENCES

1. Annual Cosmetic Surgery National Data Bank Statistics, American Society for Aesthetic Plastic Surgery, 2000–2007.
2. Kesselring UK. Regional fat aspiration for body contouring. Plast Reconstr Surg 1983;72(5):610–9.
3. Kesselring UK, Meyer R. A suction curette for removal of excessive local deposits of subcutaneous fat. Plast Reconstr Surg 1978;62(2):305–6.
4. Klein JA. Anesthesia for liposuction in dermatologic surgery. J Dermatol Surg Oncol 1988;14(10):1124–32.
5. Klein JA. Tumescent technique for local anesthesia improves safety in large-volume liposuction. Plast Reconstr Surg 1993;92(6):1085–98.
6. Zocchi ML. Ultrasonic liposculpturing. Aesthetic Plast Surg 1992;16:287–98.
7. Maxwell GP, Gingrass MK. Ultrasound-assisted lipoplasty: a clinical study of 250 consecutive patients. Plast Reconstr Surg 1998;101(1):189–202.
8. Zocchi ML. Ultrasonic-assisted lipectomy. Adv Plast Reconstr Surg 1995;11: 197–221.
9. Silberg BN. The technique of external ultrasound-assisted lipoplasty. Plast Reconstr Surg 1998;101(2):552.
10. Fodor PB, Vogt PA. Power-assisted lipoplasty (PAL): a clinical pilot study comparing PAL to traditional lipoplasty (TL). Aesthetic Plast Surg 1999;23(6): 379–85.
11. Apfelberg DB. Laser-assisted liposuction may benefit surgeons, patients. Clin Laser Mon 1992;10(12):193–4.
12. Apfelberg DB, Rosenthal S, Hunsted JP, et al. Progress report on multicenter study of laser-assisted liposuction. Aesthetic Plast Surg 1994;18(3):259–64.
13. Apfelberg DB. Results of multicenter study of laser-assisted liposuction. Clin Plast Surg 1996;23(4):713–9.
14. Neira R, Solarte E, Reyes MA, et al. Low-level laser-assisted lipoplasty: a new technique. In: Proceedings of the World Congress on Liposuction. Dearborn (MI): 2000.

15. Neira R, Arroyave J, Ramirez H, et al. Fat Liquefaction: effect of low-level laser energy on adipose tissue. Plast Reconstr Surg 2002;110(3):912–22.
16. Neira R, Ortiz-Neira C. Low-level laser-assisted liposculpture: clinical report of 700 cases. Aesthetic Plast Surg 2002;22(5):451–5.
17. Neira R, Toledo L, Arroyave J, et al. Low-level laser-assisted liposuction: the Neira 4L technique. Clin Plast Surg 2006;33(1):117–27.
18. Blugerman G. Laser lipolysis for the treatment of localized adiposity and cellulite. In: Abstracts of the World Congress on Liposuction. Dearborn (MI): 2000.
19. Schavelzon D, Blugerman G, Goldman A, et al. Laser lipolysis. In: Abstracts of the 10th International Symposium of Cosmetic Laser Surgery. Las Vegas (NV): 2001.
20. Goldman A, Schavelzon DE, Blugerman GS. Laser lipolysis: liposuction using Nd:YAG laser. Rev Soc Bras Cir Plast 2002;17(1):17–21.
21. Goldman A, Schavelzon D, Blugerman G. Liposuction using neodymium:yttrium-aluminum-garnet laser. International Abs. Plast Reconstr Surg 2003;111(7):2497.
22. Badin AZD, Moraes LM, Gondek LB, et al. Laser lipolysis: flaccidity under control. Aesthetic Plast Surg 2002;26(5):335–9.
23. Badin AZD, Gondek LB, Garcia MJ, et al. Analysis of laser lipolysis effects on human tissue samples obtained from liposuction. Aesthetic Plast Surg 2005; 29(4):281–6.
24. Goldman A. Submental Nd:YAG laser-assisted liposuction. Lasers Surg Med 2006;38(3):181–4.
25. Ichikawa K, Miyasaka M, Tanaka R, et al. Histologic evaluation of the pulsed Nd:YAG laser for laser lipolysis. Lasers Surg Med 2005;36(1):43–6.
26. Brown SA, Rohrich RJ, Kenkel J, et al. Effect of low-level laser therapy on abdominal adipocytes before lipoplasty procedures. Plast Reconstr Surg 2004;113(6): 1796–804.
27. Kim KH, Geronemus RG. Laser lipolysis using a novel 1064 nm Nd:YAG laser. Dermatol Surg 2006;32:241–8.
28. Mordon S, Eymard-Maurin AF, Wassmer B, et al. Histologic evaluation of laser lipolysis: pulsed 1064 nm Nd:YAG laser versus CW 980 nm diode laser. Aesthetic Surg J 2007;27(3):263–8.
29. Anderson RR, Parrish JA. Selective photothermolysis: precise microsurgery by selective absorption of pulsed radiation. Science 1983;220:524–7.
30. Wollina U, Goldman A, Berger U, et al. Esthetic and cosmetic dermatology. Dermatol Ther 2008;21:118–30.
31. Goldman A, Wollina U. Subdermal Nd-YAG laser for axillary hyperhidrosis. Dermatol Surg 2008;34:756–62.
32. Goldman A, Gotkin RH, Sarnoff DS, et al. Cellulite: a new treatment approach combining subdermal Nd:YAG laser lipolysis and autologous fat transplantation. Aesthetic Surg J 2008;28(6):656–62.
33. Teimourian B, Chajchir A, Gotkin RH, et al. Semiliquid autologous fat transplantation. Adv Plast Reconstr Surg 1989;5:57–84.
34. Teimourian B, Gotkin RH. Contouring the midtrunk in overweight patients. Aesthetic Plast Surg 1989;13:145–53.
35. Teimourian B. Suction lipectomy and body sculpturing. St. Louis: C.V. Mosby Company; 1987.

Improving Outcomes in Aesthetic Facial Reconstruction

Stefan O.P. Hofer, MD, PhD, FRCS(C)[a],*, Marc A.M. Mureau, MD, PhD[b]

KEYWORDS

- Facial reconstruction • Aesthetic unit • Local flap • Free flap
- Skin cancer • Oncology

Facial reconstruction has mesmerized surgeons and the general public alike for many centuries. The earliest descriptions are of cheek flaps and later forehead flaps for nasal reconstruction done in ancient India.[1] The pioneering reconstructive work of Esser,[2] who at the beginning of the twentieth century was the first to have an understanding of vascularization in "arterial flaps," was fascinating. Current concepts of aesthetic facial reconstruction have again improved with the development of the aesthetic facial unit principle. The latest frontier in facial aesthetic reconstruction through facial transplantation is currently being challenged.

The focus of facial reconstruction has obviously always been restoration of function. With regard to aesthetics, however, facial reconstruction was considered successful when a hole was closed with a flap. Modern facial reconstruction has evolved with the help of detailed anatomic knowledge, which has made tissue transfer from local and distant sites very reliable. In recent decades, the concept of aesthetic facial reconstruction has been popularized. This concept honors the aesthetic facial units, the borders of which are made up of the transitional areas of light and shadow on the face as the facial surface changes from concave to convex (**Fig. 1**). These borders are the ideal locations to place scars. Central aesthetic facial units, such as nose or lips, can be subdivided into subunits to further refine facial reconstruction.[3] The central facial subunits (ie. nose, eyes, and lips) are ideally replaced in their entirety, if feasible, when most of the unit is lost so as to have one inconspicuous reconstructed surface.

A version of this article was previously published in the *Clinics in Plastic Surgery*, 36:2.
[a] Division of Plastic Surgery, Department of Surgery and Department of Surgical Oncology, University Health Network, University of Toronto, 200 Elizabeth Street, 8N-865, Toronto, Ontario, Canada M5G 2C4
[b] Department of Plastic and Reconstructive Surgery, Erasmus University Medical Center Rotterdam, PO Box 2040, 3000 CA Rotterdam, The Netherlands
* Corresponding author. Division of Plastic Surgery, Department of Surgery, University Health Network, 200 Elizabeth Street, 8N-865, Toronto, Ontario, Canada M5G 2C4.
E-mail address: stefan.hofer@uhn.on.ca

Perioperative Nursing Clinics 6 (2011) 147–158
doi:10.1016/j.cpen.2011.03.005
1556-7931/11/$ – see front matter © 2011 Elsevier Inc. All rights reserved.

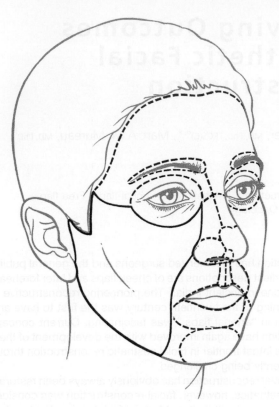

Fig. 1. Schematic representation of aesthetic units of the face.

One of the cornerstones of aesthetic facial reconstruction is meticulous defect analysis. This holds true for all reconstructive surgery in which a restoration of function is sought. In aesthetic facial reconstruction, however, additional emphasis is placed on the different aesthetic units involved as well as the quality of the tissues and the possible structural support needed by those tissues. This analysis leads to the use of the reconstructive "elevator" rather than the reconstructive "ladder," in which the flap or combination of flaps are chosen that will give the most aesthetically pleasing as well as functional outcome.[4]

From an aesthetic viewpoint, one can consider donor-site morbidity to be a result of improper scar positioning. This is largely preventable by positioning scars in the borders of the aesthetic units. For instance, when looking at a person's face, the gaze is fixed on the eyes, cheekbones, nose, and mouth. Scars on the forehead or lateral to a vertical line through the lateral canthus are less conspicuous, and therefore also have less aesthetic donor-site morbidity, even if they run through an aesthetic unit. From the functional perspective, the use of perforator flaps has greatly diminished donor-site morbidity because they save muscle function in those areas in which muscle was harvested previously to incorporate the blood supply that perfuses the overlying skin.

Aesthetic facial reconstruction is challenging and artistic. Reproducible and good outcomes can only be achieved by the use of detailed preoperative plans with possible back-up options. Proper planning is key to any good outcome. In many cases, consecutive stages need to be performed as part of the initial plan or as part of touch-ups. A perfect result will often need more than a single operation. This paper provides insight on how to prevent undesirable functional and aesthetic outcomes in facial reconstruction and gives solutions for the enhancement of functional and aesthetic outcomes using secondary procedures.

DEFECT ANALYSIS

Facial reconstruction is well beyond the period in which filling the hole or covering up the surface was a measure of success. Aesthetic facial reconstruction is only successful if normalcy and, if affected, symmetry are restored. Successful aesthetic facial reconstruction is largely dependent on the proper analysis of the defect. To properly analyze the defect, a list of the issues involved in functional impairment and the missing tissues from involved aesthetic units needs to be made. When all the requirements of the reconstruction have been identified, a plan can be made. Reconstruction of function should be the basis from which to start, after which the aesthetics of the reconstruction come in. As a general rule, aesthetic units should be reconstructed individually. For instance, a forehead flap used for nasal reconstruction should not be used to reconstruct part of a cheek because the cheek defect needs to be reconstructed separately from the nose.

FUNCTIONAL AND AESTHETIC OUTCOME ENHANCEMENT BY REGION
Forehead and Scalp

Forehead and scalp reconstruction first aims to cover exposed underlying skull bone or contents. Following successful defect coverage, the main focus of the reconstruction becomes one of a more an aesthetic nature. Successful coverage will not always result in good aesthetic outcome. Small- to medium-sized defects can be reconstructed satisfactorily using local scalp flaps (**Fig. 2**). In large defects, local tissue will not be of sufficient size to provide coverage, and free-tissue transfer will be required. The main concerns here generally are: (1) coverage that is too bulky or too thin, (2) incorrect skin color, (3) lack of hair, and (4) suboptimal scarring. In addition, sometimes a contour deficiency caused by missing bone may exist. There are a number of solutions to deal with these issues.

Suboptimal flap selection will usually result in excessive bulk after coverage of the forehead or scalp. Musculocutaneous flaps and thick fasciocutaneous flaps can result in bulky coverage. Skin on the forehead and scalp and related subcutaneous tissues are generally thinner than in most standard skin flap areas. Excising the skin paddle of a musculocutaneous flap and skin grafting the underlying muscle can thin excessive bulk of skin and subcutis. Alternatively, resection or liposuction of subcutaneous fat can further thin a flap.

When using a muscle flap with skin graft for coverage, the muscle will thin over time because it is no longer innervated. On the scalp, this will usually not be a major concern. These flaps, however, are less resilient to friction and can present with small areas of skin graft breakdown over time. On the forehead, thinning of a muscle flap can result in a skeletonized appearance, which accentuates the contour of the skull. Correction of this aesthetic problem can be solved by using reconstruction with a regional thin skin flap of appropriate skin color and texture, which, if unavailable, can be generated by flap prefabrication (**Fig. 3**).

The final skin paddle color of the flap used in a reconstruction is mostly hard to predict. Skin grafts will often change to a different color, which usually is not the color of the surrounding skin. Good results have been reported for skin grafting of the facial area using scalp skin grafts. This is a feasible option for forehead and facial skin

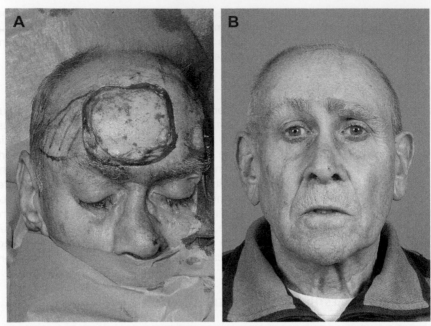

Fig. 2. Patient with defect on the forehead after radical full-thickness resection of squamous cell carcinoma. (*A*) Design of a scalp rotation flap, based on the superficial temporal and retroauricular vessels, with excision of a Burrow's triangle placing the final scar line at the superior brow line. (*B*) Final result after one operation. A large back cut and a split thickness skin graft were required on the posterior scalp to accommodate closure of the donor defect after scalp rotation.

reconstruction, but not for larger scalp reconstructions. Alternatively, skin grafting of a de-epithelialized, previously transferred, (distant) free flap using a scalp skin graft may improve skin color match.[5] An axiom states that skin flaps taken from sites closer to the face have better color match. This has not always been the authors' experience. Skin from areas that are primarily protected from the sun by clothes, like parascapular flap skin, is generally unpredictable in the way that it will color when transplanted to the facial area. For scalp reconstructions, it is less important to have an exact color match because many of these patients will wear hairpieces or wigs to cover the baldness.

Restoration of hair after scalp or forehead reconstruction can be addressed by using hair transplantation for smaller defects or eyebrows. Tissue expansion of remaining hair-bearing scalp to replace bald areas can be performed. When large hair-bearing scalp defects are present, men will have a bald head or a wig can be worn. The smaller the scalp defect, the more likely the area will be covered with a hairpiece or remaining hair as the easiest options. A simple alternative solution for eyebrow restoration can be tattooing.

Eyelids

The eyes are one of the areas of primary focus in social interaction. Eyelid defects, which cannot be closed primarily, should be reconstructed according to ocular plastic surgical principles. Eyelid reconstruction serves to prevent functional complications in this complex region and to preserve aesthetic harmony. Eyelid function, which is protection of the eye and maintaining hydration of the cornea, should be restored

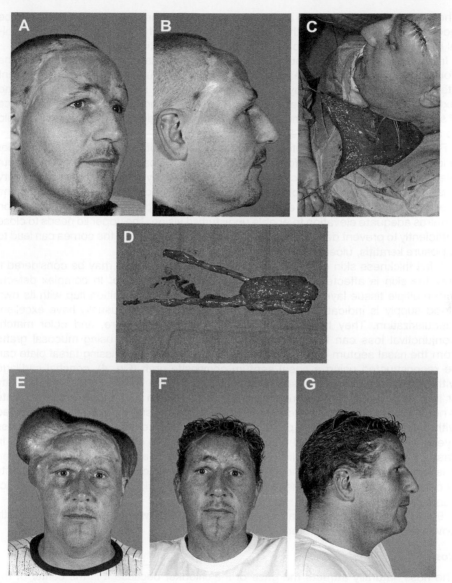

Fig. 3. Patient 9 months after the use of a rectus abdominis muscle free flap with split thickness skin graft from the thigh to reconstruct a defect after radical resection by an ENT surgeon of the outer table of the frontal bone in combination with all overlying soft tissues to treat severe sinusitis that had not resolved after more than 70 surgical attempts. (*A*) Three-quarter right view and (*B*) lateral view. Reconstruction of the forehead using an overlying skin graft was requested to improve the skeletonized appearance and the frequent breakdown of the atrophied muscle. The left-sided neck skin was prefabricated (*C*) by placing an adipofascial radial forearm free flap (*D*) under the neck skin. (*E*) At the same time, multiple tissue expanders were inserted under the scalp to restore the anterior hairline. End result after prefabricated neck skin free flap transfer and anterior hairline restoration in frontal (*F*) and lateral (*G*) view.

whenever feasible. The lateral and medial canthus and the tear duct system should be reconstructed, if affected. Without detailed knowledge of the anatomy of the periorbital region, it will not be possible to achieve a good functional and aesthetic result.

Incisions are preferably made parallel to the skin folds to minimize tension on the wound and vertical pull on the eyelid rim. Skin grafts should blend in with the recipient site. This can be achieved by using skin that has the same thickness, color, and texture. The opposite upper eyelid often makes for a good donor site. Disturbance of shape, contour, position, and symmetry of the eyelid, eyebrow, and canthus should be avoided because this will effect social interaction.

Reconstruction of eyelid defects affecting up to 30% of the total length of the upper or lower lid can usually be performed by using primary closure in layers, with or without lateral cantholysis. Any defect that is reconstructed by means other than primary closure should therefore be one that affects 30% or more of the total length of the eyelid. A normal functioning eyelid is of paramount importance. Upper lid function requires adequate elevation to enable undisturbed vision. The upper lid needs to close sufficiently to prevent dehydration of the cornea. Dehydration of the cornea can lead to exposure keratitis, ulceration, and blindness.

A full-thickness skin graft (preferably from the upper eyelid) may be considered if only the skin is affected and primary closure is not possible. In complex defects with multiple tissue layers affected, use of a regional transposition flap with its own blood supply is indicated. Flaps from the periorbital region usually have excellent vascularization. They have the appropriate thickness, texture, and color match. Conjunctival loss can be replaced with "like-for-like" tissue using mucosal grafts from the nasal septum or inner cheek. Eyelid support of the missing tarsal plate can be reconstructed using a nasal septum composite graft (**Fig. 4**), conchal cartilage with or without skin, or a tarsoconjunctival flap. If there is no severe lower-lid laxity or if most of the lower lid is not missing, reconstruction of the lower-lid tarsal plate is not always necessary, provided that a mucosal graft is sutured in tightly and covered with a local transposition flap from the upper lid. Reconstruction of full-thickness eyelid loss can be performed using a full-thickness flap of the upper or lower lid. In case of full-thickness upper-lid reconstructions, this is a good technique; however, it is generally not recommended to reconstruct full-thickness lower-eyelid defects because sacrificing part of the full-thickness upper eyelid may lead to serious functional problems.

Eyelid reconstruction has a very functional focus in which aesthetics are mostly governed by the goal of restoring symmetry.

Nose

The nose naturally attracts the gaze of the onlooker because it is the center of the facial appearance. Nasal function has to act as a guide for the reconstruction. The reconstruction has to permit unobstructed airflow for normal breathing, speech, and smell.

Nasal reconstruction is based on the principle of restoration of anatomic structural layers. The nose is divided into three main layers: the mucosal lining (inner lining), the osteocartilaginous framework (structural support), and the external soft tissue and skin (outer lining).

Inner lining reconstruction is the first step in reconstructing the nose. Many options for inner lining reconstruction are available. It is important that the inner lining is thin to prevent obstruction of the nasal passage. In addition, nasal lining needs to be well vascularized to allow insertion of structural support in the process of nasal reconstruction. Inner lining materials include skin grafts, turnover flaps, mucosal flaps, folded parts of

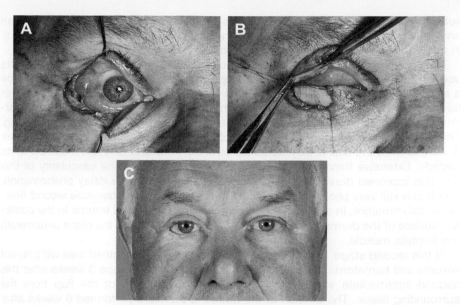

Fig. 4. Full-thickness re-resection for basal cell carcinoma of one third of the upper eyelid and one half of the lower eyelid on the right eye with destruction of the lateral canthus. (A) Reconstruction of the upper eyelid using a buccal mucosa graft for the inner lining and a musculocutaneous Tripier transposition flap for the external cover. (B) Reconstruction of the lower eyelid using a nasal composite septomucosal transposition for the inner lining and support with fixation to the lateral orbital wall and a cheek advancement flap for the external cover. (C) Result after 6 months with slightly detached lateral lower lid margin.

regional flaps, and free flaps. When secondary enhancement is needed, if initial inner lining reconstruction did not prove satisfactory, improvement of outcome mostly involves the use of local tissue rearrangement or the addition of skin grafts to add to the shortage of inner lining. Providing enough inner lining is of paramount importance during the first reconstructive procedure because correction of inner lining shortage during later stages is very hard to achieve.[6] In rare cases, the entire reconstruction has to be redone.

Structural support is vital in nasal reconstruction to maintain projection, restore the external and internal nasal valve, and allow for nasal air passage. Autologous materials such as auricular, septal, or costal cartilage are preferred materials. Structural support is not only required to replace the missing support but also to add support to previously unsupported areas such as the alar rim. This extra support is vital in most areas to withstand forces of wound contraction. In cases of secondary enhancement of structural support, the addition of extra cartilage to insufficiently supported areas (eg, columella) or unsatisfactorily projecting areas (eg, nasal tip) is generally undertaken. These cartilage grafts need to be thin to prevent too much bulk in the nose, yet strong to withstand all of the forces working on them.

The nose is given its external, three-dimensional appearance by its convex and concave surfaces. The surface contours are the basis of the nine-aesthetic subunit principle developed by Burget and Menick.[7] These contours have to be considered carefully when recreating or adapting the defect. When providing the external skin cover, scars are placed in the boundaries of these units to make them less conspicuous. Generally, it is advisable to replace the entire subunit if 50% or more of that subunit is missing. Leaving smaller areas of a remaining subunit will result in an unsightly scar across a visual plane that should not have a scar and can easily result in distortion because of trapdooring and scar contraction.

The paramedian forehead flap is the workhorse flap for nasal reconstruction. Its use is best regarded as a three-stage operation, whether it is used to resurface a single-layer nasal defect or employed in a complex, three-layer nasal reconstruction. The first operation allows for laying the basis of the reconstruction by transferring the forehead flap, which has a very reliable blood supply without any thinning. The second stage allows for fine tuning of the flap and extensive thinning at week 3. At this time, the flap is fully detached from the nose and only left attached to its pedicle. Extensive thinning is tolerated at this time because the vascularity of this flap has improved during the first 3 weeks as the result of the delay phenomenon. The flap is still very pliable and moldable at this second stage because wound healing is still immature. In addition, there has also been no surgical trauma to the posterior surface of the dermis because the flap was initially raised in the plane underneath the frontalis muscle.

At this second stage, loosely placed quilting sutures in the thinned area will prevent seroma and hematoma formation. The third stage will take place 3 weeks after this second intermediate stage. This allows for vascularization of the flap from the surrounding tissue. The division of the pedicle is therefore performed 6 weeks after the original surgery (**Fig. 5**).

For secondary enhancement of outcomes, further touch-up operations will be postponed for at least 6 months to let wound healing occur, swelling disappear, and the nose soften. The procedures undertaken at that time are usually geared toward repositioning scars into the correct aesthetic units, thinning areas of excessive bulk, improving contour through shaping of subcutaneous tissue, or adding tissue to areas of tightness or contraction. When making these secondary enhancements, old scars can be disregarded, whereas new incisions should be placed exactly at the borders of aesthetic subunits.[8]

Cheeks

The cheek lies on the periphery of an onlooker's gaze in social interaction. As such, this area of the face falls to less critical appraisal when it comes to minor details, compared with appraisal of the nose, lips, and eyes. To achieve a good result in cheek reconstruction, it is important to restore normal facial surface appearance. This can be achieved by restoring a uniform skin color and texture, and is not so much dependent on contour and outline.

From a functional perspective, there are few requirements in cheek reconstruction unless there is a very extensive defect or a deeper lesion involving the facial nerve. In those cases, either distant or free flaps may be required to cover underlying structures or fill up cavities, or facial nerve repair or reconstruction is indicated.

In general, cheek defects that are not amenable to primary closure are preferably reconstructed using local tissues to prevent the color mismatch and inadequate bulk that distant tissues usually bring with them. In those cases in which only contour but no skin is lacking, the use of free-tissue transfer, local subcutaneous adipofascial flaps, or lipofilling for lesser bulk requirements can be very good options. Local flaps supplying "like-with-like" skin are either anterior-based, rotation-advancement flaps that are vascularized by the facial and submental vessels or posterior-based, rotation-advancement flaps supplied by the superficial temporal and preauricular vessels. The use of free-tissue flaps, if required, will often lead to suboptimal aesthetic outcome.[9]

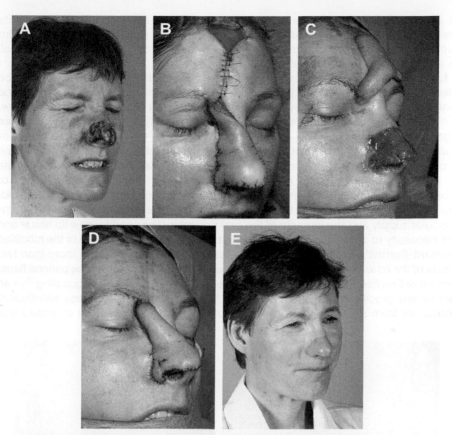

Fig. 5. (*A*) Skin defect of the nasal tip and ala, extending into the nasal dorsum and sidewall after Mohs' resection for basal cell cancer. (*B*) First stage paramedian forehead flap reconstruction. (*C*) Second stage thin lifting of paramedian forehead flap and sculpting of the nose with placement of delayed primary alar rim batten cartilage graft. (*D*) Repositioning of thin second stage paramedian forehead flap and placement of ala-defining quilting sutures. (*E*) Result one year after reconstruction.

For obtaining an optimal aesthetic cheek reconstruction result, skin coverage of the defect should ideally be reconstructed using the aforementioned local or locoregional flaps, whenever possible. As mentioned before in this article, it is important to place scars in the aesthetic unit borders if possible. In addition, improved outcome is achieved if no scars run anterior to a vertical line drawn through the lateral canthus. The transposition of cheek skin often gives a downward pull on the lower eyelid. Attention should be directed at producing very strong support and overcorrection of the position of these flaps whenever there is a chance of downward pull to prevent ectropion. Fixation of the flap to the periorbital bony tissues using drill holes or bone anchors is a very useful technique.

Lips

The lips are important from a functional as well as from an aesthetic viewpoint. They play a vital role in facilitating speech and food intake and are a focal point of the central face during social contact. All the concepts of facial reconstruction play an equally important role in reconstructive surgery of the lips. Careful defect analysis is required to assess restorative options for function and loss of aesthetics. Any abnormality resulting from asymmetry in shape or movement will be picked up. This can be from such extreme cases as complete facial nerve palsy or total lip resection to as small as a step deformity in the white roll.

Lip defects are not different from other defects in that it is important to try to replace "like" tissue with "like" tissue. Lip tissue has such a specific anatomy and appearance that it is hard to replace it in a pleasing fashion using an alternate tissue source. Smaller lip defects of up to one third of the lip can usually be closed primarily without significant problems. Slightly larger defects may require the use of a lip shave or buccal mucosal advancement flaps for vermilion reconstruction, and lip switch flaps such as the Abbe and Estlander flaps for moderate-sized (less than one half of the lip length), full-thickness lip reconstruction (**Fig. 6**). If the defect lies centrally or more laterally with involvement of the commissure and no new lip tissue is required, the Karapandzic flap provides the ideal reconstruction because it preserves the neurovascular supply and the integrity of the oral sphincter. The need for new lip tissue and the necessity to avoid microstomia are the best indications for the use of the modified Bernard-Burrow's procedures. For large lower-lip defects measuring more than two thirds of the lip without sufficient cheek tissue available to execute these perioral flaps, distant or free flaps such as a free radial forearm flap with palmaris longus sling[10] or an innervated gracilis free flap are required.[11] These flaps will give less satisfactory outcomes from a functional and aesthetic view. Patients should be educated that

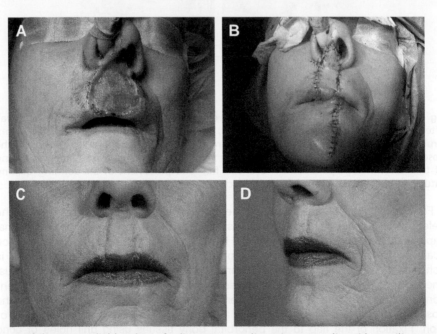

Fig. 6. Philtrum, medial borders of adjacent upper lip units, upper lip mid-vermilion, and partial columella defect after Mohs' resection for basal cell cancer. (*A*) Reconstruction of the defect after changing the defect into full-thickness defect. Bilateral medial advancement of the lateral upper lip units was performed to bring back the defect to a philtrum and columella defect. (*B*) Reconstruction of the philtrum and partial columella defect using an Abbe flap from the lower lip. (*C*) Anterior and (*D*) three-quarter view of the end result after 2 years, with an intermediate operation to separate the columella and philtrum units using thinning and quilting.

postoperative oral function can be compromised because of tightness or impaired lip sensation.

Specific considerations to improve outcomes in lip reconstruction need to be considered. The aesthetic unit lines should be marked and incorporated in the plan of reconstruction. With the Abbe flap, it is very important to design the flap in the middle of the lower lip. In this fashion, the scar will be dead center, which prevents asymmetric distortion of the lower lip. Secondary scar revisions to get the scar in the center will only give limited success. The design of the Abbe flap should allow closure of the lower lip without pull on the vermilion to prevent distortion. Abbe flaps in men need special consideration with regard to hair growth. By turning the lower lip skin upside down, the direction of hair growth is incorrect. In addition, the hair growth on the lower lip skin is often less than that on the upper lip skin. In some cases, additional hair follicle transplants at a later date can be considered.

Step deformities, which are very visible after all wounds are healed, are caused by incorrect realignment of the white roll at initial surgery. Careful realignment after full wound healing will improve the white roll appearance. The lip vermilion can be touched up during the second operation if asymmetry resulting from bulkiness across a scar exists. Careful restoration of the continuity of the orbicularis oris muscle has to be performed to prevent a whistling deformity. The continuity of the orbicularis oris muscle can be restored secondarily, if required. In the case of persistent commissural deformity, two opposing mucosal rhomboid flaps, which are transposed laterally to reconstruct the angle, may be best used. Mucosal deficiency of the vermilion may be overcome by using an anterior-based tongue flap, which is divided after 10 to 14 days,[12] or by using a facial artery musculomucosal flap.[13]

Microstomia can be particularly troublesome for patients who use dentures. They have to be instructed how to remove and insert these appliances, so that the least amount of strain is put on the lip. A splinting device may be used for several months to treat microstomia.

SUMMARY

Functional and aesthetic outcome enhancement of facial reconstruction is a very challenging discipline. It is important not only to have a thorough understanding of the functional anatomy of the area that requires reconstruction but also be aware of the aesthetic and anthropometric properties of the area involved. The surface anatomy as we visually perceive our fellow humans during social interaction needs to be recreated in a fashion so that asymmetry and scarring do not distract us. Only with a continuous quest for perfection and an open mind will we be able to improve our results.

REFERENCES

1. McDowell F. The classic reprint. Ancient ear-lobe and rhinoplastic operations in India. Plast Reconstr Surg 1969;43(5):515–22.
2. Esser JFS. Artery flaps. Reprint of 1932 book. Rotterdam, The Netherlands: Erasmus Publishing; 2003.
3. Menick FJ. Facial reconstruction with local and distant tissue: the interface of aesthetic and reconstructive surgery. Plast Reconstr Surg 1998;102(5):1424–33.
4. Gottlieb LJ, Krieger LM. From the reconstructive ladder to the reconstructive elevator [Editorial]. Plast Reconstr Surg 1994;93(7):1503–4.
5. Walton RL, Cohn AB, Beahm EK. Epidermal overgrafting improves coloration in remote flaps and grafts applied to the face for reconstruction. Plast Reconstr Surg 2008;121(5):1606–13.

6. Mureau MAM, Moolenburgh SE, Levendag PC, et al. Aesthetic and functional outcome following nasal reconstruction. Plast Reconstr Surg 2007;120(5): 1217–27.
7. Burget GC, Menick FJ. The subunit principle in nasal reconstruction. Plast Reconstr Surg 1985;76(2):239–47.
8. Menick FJ. A 10-year experience in nasal reconstruction with the three-stage forehead flap. Plast Reconstr Surg 2002;109(6):1839–55.
9. Mureau MAM, Posch NAS, Meeuwis CA, et al. Anterolateral thigh flap reconstruction of large external facial skin defects: a follow-up study on functional and aesthetic recipient- and donor-site outcome. Plast Reconstr Surg 2005;115(4): 1077–86.
10. Carroll CM, Pathak I, Irish J, et al. Reconstruction of total lower lip and chin defects using the composite radial forearm–palmaris longus tendon free flap. Arch Facial Plast Surg 2000;2(1):53–6.
11. Ninkovic M, Spanio di Spilimbergo S, Ninkovic M. Lower lip reconstruction: introduction of a new procedure using a functioning gracilis muscle free flap. Plast Reconstr Surg 2007;119(5):1472–80.
12. Jackson IT. Local flaps in head and neck reconstruction. 2nd edition. St. Louis (MO): QMP Publishers; 2007.
13. Pribaz JJ, Meara JG, Wright S, et al. Lip and vermilion reconstruction with the facial artery musculomucosal flap. Plast Reconstr Surg 2000;105(3):864–72.

The Physiology of Wound Healing: Injury Through Maturation

Paige Teller, MD[a], Therese K. White, MD[b],*

KEYWORDS

- Wound healing • Skin physiology • Soft tissue injury
- Coagulation cascade • Fibroplasias

The physiology of wound healing is repeatedly described in medical literature. Most classic descriptions of wound healing consist of three phases: inflammation, proliferation, and maturation. However, the three phases of wound healing are not discrete events. The true complexity of healing evolves with increasing knowledge of cellular interactions and inflammatory mediators. The stages of wound healing occur both sequentially and simultaneously. Several variations exist in the recent literature, trying to create a framework for the molecular biology and cellular physiology of the healing process. The following description of wound healing provides a general summary of the events, cellular components, and influential mediators of wound healing over time.

INJURY

The initiation of healing starts with the creation of a wound. A wound is defined as an injury to the body that typically involves laceration or breaking of a membrane and damage to the underlying tissues.[1] Injury can occur from any number of mechanical or thermal forces that lead to disruption of the skin and damage to the connective tissue and vasculature. Bleeding ensues along with exposure of collagen, endothelium, and intravascular and extravascular proteins. This environment serves as a stimulus for hemostasis.

HEMOSTASIS

The resolution of injury begins with hemostasis. Vasoconstriction and clot formation lead to cessation of bleeding. Hemostasis is achieved through the activation of platelets and the coagulation cascade.

A version of this article was previously published in *Surgical Clinics*, 89:3.
[a] Surgical Oncology, Emory University, 1365c Clifton Road NE, Atlanta, GA 30322, USA
[b] Plastic & Hand Surgical Associates, 244 Western Avenue, South Portland, ME 04106, USA
* Corresponding author. Plastic & Hand Surgical Associates, 244 Western Avenue, South Portland, Maine 04106.
E-mail address: twhite@plasticandhand.com

Perioperative Nursing Clinics 6 (2011) 159–170
doi:10.1016/j.cpen.2011.04.001
1556-7931/11/$ – see front matter © 2011 Elsevier Inc. All rights reserved.

Vasoconstriction

Contraction of the smooth muscle within the endothelium is the first response to vessel injury. Reflexive vasoconstriction occurs before activation of platelets and coagulation. The endothelium of damaged vessels produces its own vasoconstrictor, endothelin. Other mediators for vasoconstriction are derived from circulating catecholamines (epinephrine), the sympathetic nervous system (norepinephrine), and the release of prostaglandins from injured cells.[2] Coagulation and platelet activation contribute additional stimuli for vasoconstriction through the following mediators: bradykinin, fibrinopeptides, serotonin, and thromboxane A2.

Coagulation Cascade

The coagulation cascade is made up of two converging pathways: extrinsic and intrinsic. The extrinsic coagulation pathway is an essential pathway for normal thrombus formation. It is initiated by exposed tissue factor on the subendothelial surface.[2] Tissue factor binds to factor VII and leads to the subsequent activation of factors IX and X. The intrinsic pathway is not essential to coagulation. As suggested by name, all components of the pathway are intrinsic to the circulating plasma.[3] Initiation of the intrinsic pathway is through the autoactivation of factor XII. Factor XII has the unique ability to change shape in the presence of negatively charged surfaces.[4] Factor XII, in its active form, is a stimulus for the activation of factors XI, IX, VIII, and X. Although each pathway has a distinct trigger, both lead to the activation of factor X and the production of thrombin. Thrombin serves two important roles in clot formation: a catalyst for the conversion of fibrinogen to fibrin and an initiator for platelet activation **(Fig. 1)**.[5]

Platelets Adherence, Aggregation, and Degranulation

Platelets are the first cells to respond in wound healing. Activated platelets contribute to hemostasis through the process of adherence, aggregation, and degranulation. The presence of platelets at the site of injury is stimulated by exposed collagen and

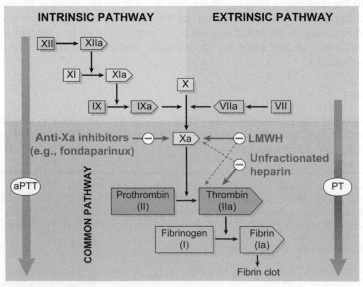

Fig. 1. Intrinsic and extrinsic coagulation pathways.

thrombin. Collagen within the subendothelial matrix comes in contact with blood flow, leading to the adhesion of circulating platelets. Platelet adherence is achieved through interactions between platelet glycoproteins VI and collagen. Additional interactions occur between platelet glycoprotein Ib-V-IX complex and collagen-bound von Willebrand's factor. Platelet integrins play a supportive role in the adherence of platelets to collagen, von Willebrand's factor, fibrinogen, and other platelets.[5]

As mentioned above, tissue factor activates the extrinsic coagulation pathway leading to the production of thrombin. Thrombin is an independent initiator of platelet activation. Thrombin interacts with a receptor on the platelet surface (Par1) and leads to the release of ADP, serotonin, and thromboxane A2.[5] These substances enhance platelet aggregation. Thromboxane A2 and serotonin also act as potent mediators of vasoconstriction.[3] Platelet aggregation in the environment of the fibrin matrix forms a clot.

Thrombus prevents ongoing bleeding, establishes a protective barrier, and provides a reservoir for substances released by platelet degranulation. Degranulation involves the release of numerous cytokines, growth factors, and matrix proteins stored within platelet alpha granules. These substances promote a variety of cellular and extracellular mechanisms important to hemostasis as well as several other stages of wound healing: matrix deposition, chemotaxis, cell proliferation, angiogenesis, and remodeling (**Table 1**).[3,6]

INFLAMMATION

Achievement of hemostasis leads to the immediate onset of inflammation. Inflammation is evident through the physical signs of erythema, heat, edema, and pain. On a cellular level, inflammation represents vessel dilation, increased vascular permeability, and leukocyte recruitment to the site of injury. Two leukocyte populations sequentially dominate the inflammatory events of wound healing: neutrophils and macrophages. Both provide the critical function of wound debridement, whereas the latter also promotes ongoing cellular recruitment and activation necessary for subsequent steps in wound healing (**Fig. 2**).

Vasodilation and Increased Permeability

The establishment of vasoconstriction for hemostasis lasts only minutes before several factors stimulate the reverse response of vasodilation. Vasodilation is mediated by the presence of kinins, histamine, prostaglandins, and leukotrienes.[2] Vascular dilation increases blood flow to the wound, resulting in the characteristic inflammatory signs of erythema and heat. Increased flow also hastens the delivery of circulating cells and mediators to the site of injury. As vessels dilate, gaps form between the endothelial cells, increasing vascular permeability. Many of the same mediators of vasodilation (prostaglandins and histamine) also stimulate increased vascular permeability. Vasodilation in conjunction with increased permeability allows the transport of intravascular fluid, protein, and cellular components into the extravascular space. The extravasation fluid and migration of cells result in wound edema.

Leukocyte Migration and Chemotaxis

Although plasma passively leaks between endothelial gaps and proteins adhere to the wound matrix, leukocytes undergo the active process of diapedesis to enter the wound. Selectins provide weak adherence between leukocytes and the endothelium of capillaries. Stronger bonds are created between leukocytes, surface integrins, and intercellular adhesion molecules on the endothelial surface.[2] Cell migration from the endothelial surface into the extravascular space of the wound is mediated by

Table 1
Platelet alpha granule components and their role in wound healing

Adhesion Glycoproteins	Proteoglycans	Hemostasis Factors & Cofactors	Cellular Mitogens	Protease Inhibitors	Miscellaneous
• Fibronectin	• PF4	• Fibrinogen	• PDGF	• α_2-Macroglobulin	• IgG, IgA, IgM
• Vitronectin	• βTG	• Factor V, VII, XI, XII	• TGF-β	• α_2-Antitrypsin	• Albumin
• Thrombospondin	• Serglycin	• Kininogens	• ECGF	• PDCI	• GPIa/multimerin
• vWF	• HRGP	• Protein S	• EGF	• α_2-Antiplasmin	
		• Plasminogen	• VEGF/VPF	• PAI1	
			• IGF	• TFPI	
			• Interleukin-β	• α_2-PI	
				• PIXI	
				• PN-2/APP	
				• C1 inhibitor	

Data from Rendu F, Brihard-Bohn B. The platelet release reaction: granules' constituents, secretion and functions. Platelets 2001;12:261–73.

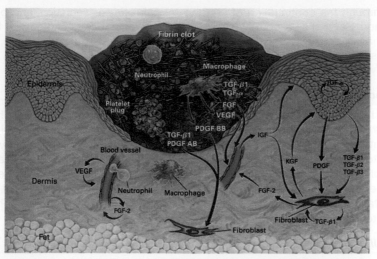

Fig. 2. Inflammatory phase day 3. (*From* Singer AJ, Clark RAF. Mechanisms of disease: Cutaneous wound healing. N Engl J Med 1999;341:739; with permission. Copyright © 1999, Massachusetts Medical Society.)

numerous chemical factors and is known as chemotaxis. Chemotactic agents can include complement factors, histamine, bacterial products, prostaglandins, leukotrienes, and growth factors. These substances recruit neutrophils, macrophages, and lymphocytes to the site of inflammation.

Neutrophils

Neutrophils are the first subset of leukocytes to enter the wound. Stimulated by prostaglandins, complement, IL-1, tumor necrosis factor alpha (TNF-α), transforming growth factor-beta TGF-β, PF4, and bacterial products, neutrophils arrive at the injury site in large numbers within 24 to 48 hours after wounding.[3–5] At this time point, neutrophils can make up 50% of all cells present within the wound. The primary functions of neutrophils are to defend the wound from bacteria and remove tissue debris. Neutrophils release several types of proteolytic enzymes, breaking down bacteria and extracellular matrix within the site of injury. Protease inhibitors protect tissue not involved in the inflammatory process. Degraded bacterial and matrix debris are removed from the wound by neutrophil phagocytosis. In addition to proteases, neutrophils produce reactive oxygen free radicals that combine with chlorine to make the wound less hospitable to bacteria.[7] The secondary role of neutrophils is to perpetuate the early phase of the inflammatory process through the excretion of cytokines.[3] One cytokine of particular importance is TNF-α. TNF-α amplifies neutrophil chemotaxis and stimulates macrophage, keratinocyte, and fibroblast expression of growth factors needed in angiogenesis and collagen synthesis. Neutrophils do not directly contribute to collagen deposition or wound strength.[3] In time, neutrophils are eliminated from the wound by either apoptosis or macrophage phagocytosis.

Macrophages

At 48 to 96 hours after wounding, the predominant leukocyte within a wound is the macrophage. Derived from extravasated monocytes, macrophages are essential to wound healing. They perform diverse tasks throughout both the inflammatory and proliferative phases of wound healing. Macrophages, like neutrophils, remove wound debris through the continuation of phagocytosis, proteases secretion, and bacterial sterilization. Serving as a primary source of numerous cytokines and growth factors, macrophages are necessary to support cellular recruitment and activation, matrix synthesis, angiogenesis, and remodeling. Unlike neutrophils, macrophages remain within a wound until healing is complete (**Table 2**).

T Lymphocytes

Attracted to the site of injury by interleukin-2 (IL-2) and other factors, T lymphocytes populate the wound to a lesser degree than macrophages. By week 2, lymphocytes represent the predominant leukocyte cell type within the wound. Lymphocytes are thought to be critical to the inflammatory and proliferative phases of repair. In addition to providing cellular immunity and antibody production, lymphocytes act as mediators within the wound environment through the secretion of lymphokines and direct cell-to-cell contact between lymphocytes and fibroblasts. The details of how lymphocytes contribute to healing are not fully understood.

Mast Cells

Another leukocyte recruited during inflammation is the mast cell. Mast cells can achieve a five-fold increase in number at the site of injury. Granules within the mast cells contain histamine, cytokine (TNF-α), prostaglandins, and protease. Degranulation leads to enhanced vascular permeability, cellular activation, collagen deposition, and remodeling (**Fig. 3**).

PROLIFERATION

The events of inflammation lead to wound debridement. Once debrided, wound healing enters a constructive phase of repair. This stage of wound healing is referred to as the proliferative phase. Proliferation takes place around postinjury days 4 through 12. During this time period, fibroblasts, smooth muscle cells, and endothelial cells infiltrate the wound as epithelial cells begin to cover the site of injury. In concert, these cells reestablish tissue continuity through matrix deposition, angiogenesis, and epithelialization.[3]

Fibroplasia and Myofibroblasts

Fibroblasts are one of the last cell populations to enter the wound. They are mobilized to the site of injury by products of the cell lines that came before them. The first signals for fibroblast recruitment comes from platelet-derived products: platelet-derived growth factor (PDGF), insulin-like growth factor (IGF-1), and TGF-β. The maintenance of fibroblasts within the wound is achieved through paracrine and autocrine signals. Macrophages and fibroblasts release numerous growth factors and cytokines that contribute to fibroblast migration: fibroblast growth factor (FGF), IGF-1, Vascular endothelial growth factor (VEGF), IL-1, IL-2, IL-8, PDGF, TGF-α, TGF-β, and TNF-α.[8,9] Of these substances, PDGF is the most potent chemotactic and mitogenic factor for fibroblasts and their progenitor smooth muscle cells.[3] Fibroblasts that migrate from surrounding tissue to the wound edge are activated by PDGF and endothelial growth factor (EGF) to proliferate and begin synthesizing collagen. Additionally, these fibroblasts are capable of producing matrix metalloproteinases (MMP). Secretion of MMPs allows for the degradation of the matrix obstructive to fibroblast migration.[2] There is a second population of fibroblasts that reside within the wound. Mediated by TGF-β, these "wound fibroblasts" differ from the fibroblasts that migrate from surrounding tissue. They proliferate less, synthesize more collagen, and transform

Table 2
Macrophage activity and mediators in wound healing

Phagocytosis & Bacterial Stasis	Debridement	Cellular Recruitment & Activation	Matrix Synthesis	Angiogenesis
• Oxygen free radicals • Nitric oxide	• Collagenase • Elastase • Matrix metalloproteinase	• Growth factors: PDGF, TGF-β, EGF, IGF • Cytokines: TNF-α, IL-1, IL-6 • Fibronectin	• Growth factors: PDGF, TGF-β, EGF • Cytokines: TNF-α, IL-1, IFN-γ • Enzymes: arginase, collagenase • Prostaglandins • Nitric oxide	• Growth factors: EGF, VEGF • Cytokines: TNF-α • Nitric oxide

Data from Diegelmann RF. Cellular and biochemical aspects of normal wound healing: an overview. The Journal of Urology 1997;157(1):298–302.

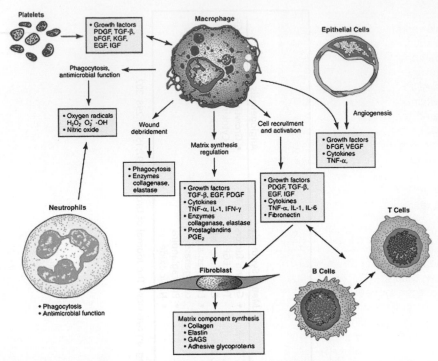

Fig. 3. Wound cells and their products: (*Adapted from* Witte MB, Barbul A. General principles of wound healing. Surg Clin North Am 1997;77:513).

into myofibroblasts involved in matrix contraction. Fibroplasia is regulated by substances that inhibit fibroblast recruitment and mitogenesis: interferon-inducible protein (IP-10), interferons, and PF4.[10]

Matrix Deposition

In addition to mediating fibroplasia, PDGF and TGF-β play important roles in matrix deposition. Both of these growth factors stimulate the fibroblast production of a provisional matrix. The matrix consists of fibroblast-derived collagen monomer, proteoglycans, and fibronectin. Together these substances reestablish the continuity of connective tissue between the wound edges. As the matrix is created, TGF-β also functions to provide structural stability though decreasing protease activity, increasing tissue inhibitors of metalloproteinase, and augmenting production of cell adhesion proteins.[10,11]

Collagen and Proteoglycan Synthesis

Collagen, the most abundant protein in the body, exists in at least 20 subtypes.[12] Two subtypes are important to wound repair. Type I collagen predominates the extracellular matrix of intact skin. Type III collagen, present in lesser amounts in undamaged skin, becomes more principal in the process of wound healing. Collagen synthesis begins hours after wounding, but it does not become significant until roughly 1 week postinjury. The activation of fibroblast to synthesize collagen is derived from growth factors and the metabolic environment within the wound. Collagen gene expression is mediated by promoter-binding sites for corticoids, TGF-β, and retinoids.

Increasing concentrations of lactate or the hypoxic environment within the wound can also stimulate collagen gene transcription and processing.[7] Lactate converts NAD+ to nicotinamide adenine dinucleotide (NADH). This depletes the availability of NAD+ to be converted into adenosine diPhosphate ribosome (ADPR). ADPR is an inhibitor of collagen mRNA transcription and other steps of collagen transport. Thus, a reduction in ADPR leads to increase in collagen mRNA synthesis. Collagen transcription occurs within the nucleus of the fibroblast. The transcribed mRNA is processed and translated by ribosomes. The resultant polypeptide chain has a repeated triplet pattern with a praline or lysine in the second position and a glycine in every third position. This protocollagen is roughly 1000 amino acids in size. On entering the endoplasmic reticulum, the protocollagen undergoes hydroxylation and glycosylation. The process of hydroxylation requires the presence of cofactors (oxygen and iron), cosubstrate (a-ketogultarate), and an electron donor (ascorbic acid).[3] Hydrogen bond formation is altered in the hydroxylated and glycosylated protocollagen chain, resulting in an a-helix. Protocollagen becomes procollagen as three a-helical chains wrap together in a right-handed superhelix. Procollagen is packaged within the Golgi apparatus and exported into the extracellular matrix. Within the extracellular space, a procollagen peptidase cleaves the ends of the chains, allowing for further cross-linking and polymerization. The covalent bond formation increases the strength of the resulting collagen monomer.[3]

In addition to collagen, fibroblasts produce and secrete glycosaminoglycans. Typically, glycosaminoglycans couple with protein to become sulfated, polysaccharide chains known as proteoglycans. Proteoglycans are thought to be a primary constituent of the "ground substance" of granulation tissue. As the collagen matrix replaces the fibrin clot, proteoglycans may provide a supportive role for the assembly of collagen fibrils.

Angiogenesis

Vascular damage incurred through wounding undergoes the restorative process of angiogenesis. Angiogenesis begins within the first 1 to 2 days after vessel disruption and can become visibly evident by approximately 4 days postinjury. Endothelial cells from intact venules migrate from the periphery to the edge of the wound. Replication follows migration and new capillary tubules form. Integrins (alpha$_v$, beta$_3$) upregulate on the endothelial cell surface, allowing for enhanced adhesion.[13–15] Proteolytic degradation of the surrounding wound matrix facilitates the advancement of new vessels across the wound.[13] In closed wounds, tubules from opposing edges quickly coalesce to revascularize the wound. Unlike closed wounds, the new capillary tubules of an unclosed wound merge with the adjacent vessel growing in the same direction, which contributes to the formation of granulation tissue.[7] The events of angiogenesis are regulated by a milieu of growth hormones (TNF-α, TGF-β, VEGF, FGF, PDGF) derived from platelets, macrophages, and damaged endothelial cells.[13] In addition to these mediators, the metabolic environment of the wound influences angiogenesis. Increased lactate along with decreased pH and oxygen tension contribute to a reduction in NAD+, an inhibitor of angiogenesis (**Fig. 4**).

Epithelialization

Much like angiogenesis, restoration of the epithelium begins early in healing, but it is not readily apparent until several days after wounding. Epithelialization reestablishes the external barrier that minimizes fluid losses and bacterial invasion. The process of epithelialization begins with epidermal thickening along wound edges.[3] Basal cells at the margins of the wound elongate.[2] Attachments between hemidesmosomes of

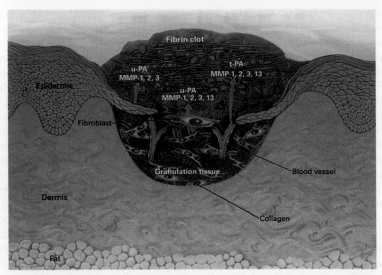

Fig. 4. Reepithelialization and neovascularization day 5. (*From* Singer AJ, Clark RAF. Mechanisms of disease: Cutaneous wound healing. N Engl J Med 1999;341:739; with permission. Copyright © 1999, Massachusetts Medical Society.)

the basal cells and the laminin of the basal lamina are broken down, allowing the cells to migrate. Migratory movements are facilitated by the expression of new integrins at the cell surface. Intracellular production and contraction of actinomycin also contribute to the forward progression of cells across the wound.[13] Epithelial cells are capable of secreting MMP to breakdown fibrin in the course of their migration. The movement of basal cells parallels the direction of collagen fiber orientation within the wound, a process termed "contact guidance."[2] Epithelial cells will continue to migrate and proliferate until they come in contact with epithelial cells traveling from other directions. Contact inhibition signals the epithelial cells to cease their migratory effort.[2] A new monolayer of epithelium is created over the site of injury. Cells in this layer differentiate to take on a less elongated and more cuboidal or basal cell appearance. Hemidesmosomes bind once again to the basement membrane, reattaching these basal-like cells. Subsequent cellular proliferation leads to reestablishment of a multilayer epidermis.[2] The events of epithelialization are influenced by intercellular signals, growth factors, and the metabolic environment within the wound. Low oxygen tension within the wound leads to increased production of TGF-β. TGF-β helps keep epithelial cells from differentiating, allowing for ongoing migration and mitogenesis. TGF-α and keratinocyte growth factor (KGF) more directly stimulate cellular replication. Conversely, moisture and higher oxygen tension support the differentiation of epithelial cells to complete the later events of epithelialization.[7]

MATURATION AND REMODELING

In summary, the events of repair began with hemostasis and creation of a fibrin-fibronectin clot. Thrombus degradation followed with the arrival of inflammatory neutrophils and macrophages. Fibroplasia provided the ground substance made up of glycosaminoglycans, proteoglycans, and other proteins to support collagen deposition. New vessels navigated through this matrix as the new epithelium traversed the wound. The final events of repair remain collagen remodeling and strengthening.

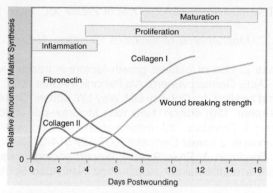

Fig. 5. Graph: relative amounts of matrix synthesis/Days postwound healing. (*Adapted from* Witte MB, Barbul A. General principles of wound healing. Surg Clin North Am 1997;77:513.)

Collagen Maturation

The last and longest event of wound healing is collagen maturation, starting 1 week postinjury and continuing for any where from 12 to 18 months. During this time period, the collagen matrix continually undergoes reabsorption and deposition to remodel and strengthen the wound. The initial collagen matrix differs in content and organization from that of uninjuried connective tissue. Intact tissue is composed of 80% to 90% type I collagen and 10% to 20% type III collagen. In contrast, the collagen matrix of an early wound consists of 30% type III collagen. The higher proportion of type III collagen contributes to a weaker matrix. Additionally, collagen fibrils within the matrix are more heavily glycosylated and thinner. These fibers are in a parallel orientation and do not interlace. At 1 week, the matrix strength is 3% of unwounded tissue. Collage-nases and proteases cleave and degrade these early collagen fibrils.[11] This process is countered ongoing by collagen deposition. Newly deposited collagen increases in thickness, strength, and organization. Lysyl oxidase promotes cross-linking between fibrils.[11] With time, the ratio of type I to type II collagen approximates that of intact connective tissue.[7] By 3 weeks, the tissue strength increases to 30%. After 3 months, the tissue achieves a maximum of 80% its original strength **(Fig. 5)**.[10]

Healed wounds are not capable of completely restoring the quality structure of intact tissue. The ability to closely approximate uninjured tissue is heavily dependent on size, depth, location and type of wound, as well as the nutritional status, wound care, and overall health of the patient.

An understanding of the basic science of wound healing is crucial to the clinician. Limitless intrinsic and extrinsic patient factors affect each step of this complex process. By understanding the underlying biology, we can significantly influence our patients' ability to heal.

REFERENCES

1. Merriam-Webster Dictionary. Available at: http://www.merriam-webster.com.
2. Lawrence WT. Wound healing biology and its application to wound management. In: O'Leary JP, Capota LR, editors. Physiologic basis of surgery. 2nd edition. Philadelphia: Lippincott Williams & Wilkins; 1996. p. 118–35.
3. Efron DE, Chandrakanth A, Park JE, et al. Wound healing. In: Brunicardi C, Andersen DK, Billiar TR, editors. Schwartz's principles of surgery. 8th edition. New York: McGraw-Hill; 2005.

4. Schmaier A. The elusive physiologic role of Factor XII. J Clin Invest 2008;118: 3006–9.

5. Furie B, Furie C. Mechanisms of thrombus formation. N Engl J Med 2008;359: 938–49.

6. Rozman P, Bolta Z. Use of platelet growth factors in treating wounds and soft-tissue injuries. Acta Dermatovenerol Alp Panonica Adriat 2007;16(4):156–65.

7. Hunt TK. Wound healing. In: Doherty GM, Way LW, editors. Current surgical diagnosis and treatment. 12th edition. New York: McGraw-Hill; 2006.

8. Eming SA, Krieg T, Davidson JM. Inflammation in wound repair: molecular and cellular mechanisms. J Invest Dermatol 2007;127:514–21.

9. Schugart RC, Friedman A, Zhao R, et al. Wound angiogenesis as a function of oxygen tension: a mathematical model. Proc Natl Acad Sci U S A 2008;105: 2628–33.

10. Broughton G, et al. The basic science of wound healing. Plast Reconstr Surg 2006;117(7S):12S–34S.

11. Diegelmann RF. Cellular and biochemical aspects of normal wound healing: an overview. J Urol 1997;157(1):298–302.

12. Adams CA, Biffi WL, Cioffi WG. Wounds, bites and stings. In: Feliciano DV, Mattox KL, Moore EE, editors. Trauma. 6th edition. New York: McGraw-Hill; 2008.

13. Martin P. Wound healing – aiming for perfect skin regeneration. Science 1997; 276:76–81.

14. Werner S, Grose R. Regulation of wound healing by growth factors and cytokines. Physiol Rev 2003;83:835–70.

15. Gillitzer R, Geobeler M. Chemokines in cutaneous wound healing. J Leukoc Biol 2001;69:513–21.

Skin Flaps

Mary Tschoi, MD[a], Erik A. Hoy, BS[b], Mark S. Granick, MD[a],*

KEYWORDS

• Skin flap • Skin transposition • Reconstructive surgery

Open wounds, particularly around the face, often require complicated techniques for optimal closure. The approach to the closure of the complicated wound depends largely on the nature of the wound, including the location and size of the defect, the functional outcome after closure, the medical comorbidities of the patient, neighboring structures, and whether the defect is secondary to a malignancy or trauma. The goals of wound management are optimal aesthetic outcome, preservation of function, and patient satisfaction.

The authors briefly review basic skin closure options and discuss use of skin flaps, particularly of the head and neck region.

HISTORY OF SKIN FLAPS

The earliest documented surgical intervention to rebuild a complicated defect occurred in India in 700 BC. Sushruta published a description of a forehead flap for nasal reconstruction. This information was not available to Western medicine until the late 1700s, when a British surgeon noted the technique still used in India and wrote a brief description in *Gentleman's Quarterly*.

Independently, the Italians developed delayed flaps, tube flaps, and flap transfers by using the upper inner arm skin to reconstruct a nose. This technique was published by Tagliacozzi in the 1500s. In modern medicine, the use of local flaps to repair facial defects began to evolve during the mid-1800s. A variety of flaps were used, but the blood supply and the dynamics of the surgery were not well understood. Harold Gilles popularized tube flaps and flap delays and initiated an interest in reconstructive surgery after World War I.[1]

Local skin flaps, such as those described in this article, were primarily refined in the 1950s in Europe and the United States by the second generation of plastic surgeons. Ian MacGregor[2,3] recognized the importance of an axial blood supply in flap surgery in the 1970s. Plastic surgeons have subsequently redefined cutaneous blood supply.

A version of this article was previously published in *Surgical Clinics* 89:3.
[a] Division of Plastic Surgery, Department of Surgery, New Jersey Medical School-UMDNJ, 90 Bergen Street, Suite 7200, Newark, NJ 07103, USA
[b] New Jersey Medical School-UMDNJ, 185 South Orange Avenue, Newark, NJ 07103, USA
* Corresponding author.
E-mail address: mgranickmd@umdnj.edu

Perioperative Nursing Clinics 6 (2011) 171–186
doi:10.1016/j.cpen.2011.04.002
1556-7931/11/$ – see front matter © 2011 Elsevier Inc. All rights reserved.

Countless vascularized flaps have since been developed. The skin flaps discussed in this article are primarily random flaps.[1-3]

PREOPERATIVE PLANNING AND CONSIDERATIONS

For each patient, a medical history encompassing smoking, peripheral vascular disease, atherosclerosis, diabetes mellitus, steroids, and previous surgeries should be elicited, because of the effects of these factors on wound healing and skin perfusion.

In managing the excisional defect, the surgeon must first assess the size and depth of the wound, as well as the nature of any exposed underlying internal anatomy. A defect containing exposed bone, nerves, or blood vessels usually necessitates a more advanced closure than would a less complicated wound.

The quality of the surrounding skin is also of great importance. Skin quality may vary from young, tight, and elastic to aged, dry, and lax. The wrinkled skin of an older patient produces less obvious scarring and offers the opportunity to conceal scars within skin tension lines. Skin that is more oily or heavily pigmented generally yields a less favorable scar. Color match is also of importance in deciding on the flap donor site. The presence of actinic damage, skin diseases, and premalignant satellite lesions should be considered. Finally, location is of major concern. Defects adjacent to critical anatomic structures, such as the eyelids, the nares, the oral commissure, and the external auditory meatus, must be reconstructed so as to avoid distorting the anatomy unique to those areas. Any alteration of these surrounding landmarks may compromise functional and aesthetic results. Previous surgical incisions and traumatic scars should also be assessed before the closure of the defect is designed.

Well-planned and -executed reconstruction of facial defects is particularly important because of the visibility of the result and the potential for functional deficits. However, the principles presented here may be applied to the management of all complicated wounds.

In the repair of facial tumor defects, the most important consideration is the management of the tumor. Incompletely excised tumor should not be covered by a flap. Skin adjacent to a tumor resection margin should not be turned over to line the nasal cavity or any other site where it will be difficult to examine. In patients who have a history of multiple or recurrent skin cancers, a strategy must be developed to allow for serial repairs. No bridges should be burned along the way. When planning a reconstruction, one must protect function first, then consider the cosmetic issues. It is crucial to discuss options with patients so that they can offer any biases that must be respected. A good-looking static repair that compromises dynamic function is unacceptable. The anatomic boundaries of the face are the allies of a good plastic surgeon. They must be respected and will be helpful in camouflaging scars.

Many defects can be treated with primary closure, secondary healing, or skin grafts. However, if, after careful assessment of the lesion, defect, and patient, the surgeon determines that the patient needs a flap for closure, he or she can apply techniques that produce the optimal aesthetic outcome.

TUMOR RESECTION

The paramount consideration in tumor excision should be the complete removal of the tumor. Although the surgeon should have a number of reconstructive options in mind, the planned reconstruction should not dictate the extent of tumor excision. The surgeon must remain open to alternative reconstructive techniques. If the defect obtained in excising the tumor cannot reasonably be reconstructed at the time of the operation, the wound should be dressed and the reconstruction reconsidered and delayed, or the patient should be referred to another surgeon specializing in these repairs. This option is clearly preferable to a suboptimal reconstruction.

BASIC SKIN CLOSURE TECHNIQUES

Undermining is performed to mobilize the tissue in areas surrounding the defect and to facilitate the draping of skin over the wound. The use of undermining allows the surgeon to move some portions of the wound and not others to avoid the distortion of nearby anatomy, such as the nasolabial fold or the oral commissure. However, because tight closures make for unsightly scars, alternatives should be considered before undermining the edges of a gaping or complicated wound. Undermining can destroy some of the options for flap repair. The reconstruction should be well planned before any undermining. In addition, the surgeon can use closure of the defect in layers to avoid any tension at the wound closure site that might result in dehiscence, wound healing problems, or widened scars.

When using elliptic skin excisions, one should make the long axis four times greater in length than the smaller axis. When an ellipse is made too short or one side of the ellipse is of unequal length, the skin may bunch at one end of the closure. This effect is known as a dog ear. In any wound, whether its sides are of equal or unequal length, the ends of the defect should be closed first to avoid unnecessary dog ears. Any redundancies can be dealt with in the middle of the wound during closure. Irregularities or pleats in the midportion of the wound generally resolve over time. Excising dog ears when they occur is simple. This excision is accomplished by extending the elliptic excision or by cutting the corner of the excision into a Burow's triangle. Alternatively, placing a small right angle or 45° bend in the affected end of the wound closure can produce a satisfactory result. Finally, a V-shaped excision of the lateral ellipse can be used, resulting in an M-plasty closure.

RECONSTRUCTIVE OPTIONS

The final outcome in any closure depends on the proper assessment of the defect and the selection of an appropriate closure technique. Primary closure involving direct approximation of the wound edges is a first option. An intermediate closure consists of approximation and closure of deeper tissue levels before final skin closure. Complex closure entails approximation and adjustment of the wound edges by means of undermining, the excision of any dog ears, or trimming of wound edges before closure. Finally, the options of skin grafting, allografting, and flap repair must be considered.

When a wound cannot be closed primarily, the options are as follows: secondary wound healing, skin grafting (discussed elsewhere), or local tissue transposition. Healing by secondary intention consists of two phenomena. The major means of size reduction of the defect is wound contracture, accompanied by re-epithelization to a lesser extent. Wound contracture may result in distortion of nearby mobile anatomic features, such as the oral commissure or the epicanthi. The contraction of scar tissue alters the orientation of the surrounding normal anatomy, which may result in an unacceptable cosmetic outcome and, more importantly, in poor function.

Healing by secondary intention is a viable option in fixed areas away from important anatomy, such as the middle of the forehead, the cheek, or the neck. In areas adjacent to important, easily deformable anatomic structures, transposition flaps are often a better wound closure approach.[4,5]

SKIN FLAP COVERAGE

Local skin flaps offer several advantages. Well-designed flaps borrow skin from areas of relative excess and transpose it to fill a defect. The skin provided is a close match in both color and texture, the donor site can be closed directly, and scar contracture is minimal. However, these flaps require experience and planning. Preliminarily drawing two or three flap design options for the defect may provide the surgeon with the best visualization of the optimal choice of flap for the particular area and defect. The choice of flap depends on the location and size of the defect, the quality of the surrounding skin, and the location of adjacent excess tissue. One should anticipate the appearance of the donor site scar and, when possible, plan to leave the scar in a natural crease line (eg, the nasolabial fold). When one raises the flap and moves it into the defect, key sutures should be applied and the overall flap position should be evaluated. If there is distortion of adjacent structures, one should reposition the key sutures and re-evaluate again for optimal position and least degree of tension. In addition, once the flap is in place and tacked down with temporary key sutures, it should be assessed for adequate perfusion. Further adjustments may be necessary. Closing the donor site first will relieve tension at the inset location. For example, closure of the Y lower limb in a V-Y flap helps push the flap to the inset position, and suturing on the bias further helps advance the flap into its recipient position. Once the final position of the flap is determined, it can be inset using the basic techniques already mentioned.

FLAP CLASSIFICATION

Flaps were first classified as random or axial by McGregor and Morgan[3] in 1973. Random flaps had no specific vascular supply. Axial flaps had an arterial and venous blood supply in the long axis of the flap. Further contributions to the classification of flaps were made by Daniel and Williams,[6] Webster,[7] Kunert,[8] and Cormack and Lamberty.[9] A random cutaneous flap's blood supply is derived from the dermal-subdermal plexuses of blood vessels, which originate from direct cutaneous, fasciocutaneous, or musculocutaneous vessels. One example is the rhomboid flap. The arterial, axial, and direct cutaneous flaps are based on septocutaneous arteries. These septocutaneous arteries come either from segmental or muscular vessels, pass through the fascia between muscles, and provide blood supply to the fascia and skin. They also give off branches to the muscle. The cutaneous portion of the septocutaneous arteries runs parallel to the skin surface and has venous comitantes running along with the artery above the muscle. An example is a forehead flap. In summary, survival of the skin flap is dependent on the vascular anatomy incorporated in the flap.[10–12]

TRANSPOSITION FLAPS

Local transposition flaps involve the movement of adjacent skin from an area of excess to the area of deficiency. These flaps involve the transfer of the flap through an arc of rotation on a pivot point in a linear axis. Regional tissue laxity and mobility are of greater importance than the precise angular/geometric measurements. In addition, the flap should be designed to fit the defect with minimal tension at the closure line, to avoid distorting the neighboring structures, and to have an adequate base to perfuse the undermined, elevated flap. The rule of thumb is that the random pattern transposition flaps should not have a linear axis longer than three times the width of the flap. Rhomboid flaps, Z-plasties, and W-plasties are variations on the transposition flap. They involve the transposition of a random skin and subcutaneous tissue flap into an adjoining defect. These flaps are designed so that the donor scar is well camouflaged. They must be meticulously designed according to the specific requirements of the reconstruction. However, transposition flaps are quick and easy for the experienced surgeon and are versatile solutions to many coverage problems. Particular areas well-suited to transposition flaps include the glabela, temple region, scalp, and lower third of the nose. Smokers and other patients with vascular compromise are at risk for flap necrosis.[13,14]

Banner Flap

The banner flap (**Fig. 1**)[15] is a transposition flap designed as a pendant of skin tangential to the edge of a round defect. The flap is elevated, and the donor site closed. The flap edges are then trimmed to fit the defect better, and the flap is inset.

   The bilobed flap (**Fig. 2**)[16–20] is a variant of the banner flap in which two adjacent segments are raised, one smaller than the other. The two flaps are oriented perpendicularly to each other. The smaller flap (usually half the diameter of the larger flap) is used to fill the larger donor site, and the small donor site is closed primarily. The original defect is then closed by means of the larger of the two lobes. The final result is the 180° rotation of excess tissue to fill the skin deficit. Bilobed flaps are most commonly used in the closure of nasal defects, particularly in the lower third, and they are a means to transfer excess adjacent skin into the area of deficiency. Defects that cannot be covered using a single transposition flap because of tension can be closed by this method. One must be aware that these curvilinear incisions will not necessarily fall into pre-existing skin folds or wrinkles.

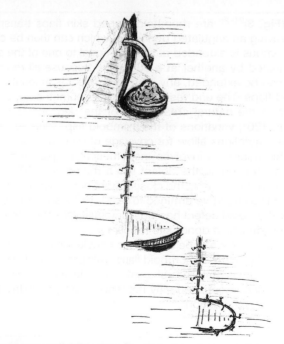

Fig. 1. The banner transposition flap. The flap is designed tangential to the defect and the donor site closed primarily.

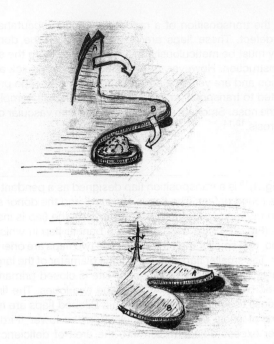

Fig. 2. The bilobed transposition flap. The primary donor flap is designed tangential to the defect, and the secondary flap is designed to be smaller and more elliptic to allow for primary closure of the secondary donor site.

Rhomboid Flap

Rhomboid flaps (**Fig. 3**)[21–25] are rhomboid-shaped skin flaps transposed into like-shaped defects leaving an angulated donor site, which can then be closed primarily. A corner of the rhombus is extended at a length equal to one of the short diagonals. This new limb is joined by another at a 60° angle. Because all rhomboids possess four corners that can be extended, any rhomboid defect is amenable to any of eight possible rhomboid flaps. The end result is a scar of geometric appearance, which is best when hidden in the natural crease lines of the skin. Although the customary angles are 60° and 120°, variations of the rhomboid flap using 30° and 150° angles are possible. These variations allow for coverage of rhomboid defects with unequal sides. Because this approach involves more meticulous planning, it is sometimes simpler to begin by converting the defect into a rhombus of 60° and 120° angles. The area of maximum tension is at the closure point of the donor site flap. The vector of maximum tension has been determined to be 20° to the short diagonal of the rhomboid defect. Every rhomboid defect has eight potential flaps for closure, and it is up to the surgeons to decide which donor site is optimal.

When a larger wound needs to be closed, the circular defect can be converted into a hexagon and closed with three rhomboid flaps. This procedure is even more complicated to plan, and it leaves a stellate-shaped scar. The scar is difficult to merge into natural crease lines and is consequently noticeable as a geometric scar. This technique should be used with caution.

Z-plasty

The Z-plasty (**Fig. 4**) is a double transposition flap that is often an appropriate option in scar revision or in the release of scar contractions. These flaps are well suited to the

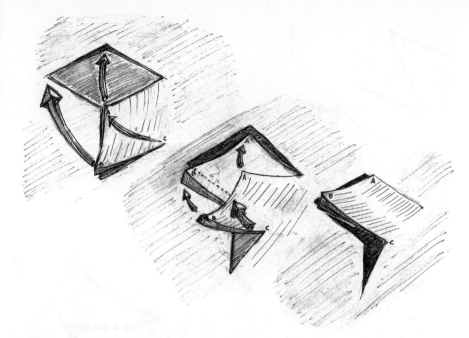

Fig. 3. The rhomboid flap.

correction of skin webs and the disruption of circumferential scars or constricting bands. Furthermore, the Z-plasty elongates the operated tissues.

The Z-plasty entails the exchange of two adjacent triangular flaps. The incision consists of a central limb and two limbs oriented to resemble a Z. All limbs are the same length to facilitate closure. The length of the central limb dictates the absolute gain in length after Z-plasty, whereas the angles chosen determine the percentage of length increase. The typical Z-plasty has 60° angles, resulting in a gain in length of 70% relative to the central limb. The angles may range from 30° to 90°, providing gains in length of 25% and 120%, respectively.[4] However, these gains are theoretic. Smaller gains are seen in practice because of restrictive skin factors. Because the Z-plasty relies on healthy adjacent skin, it is usually a poor choice for the correction of burn scar contractures. However, the gain in length granted by the Z-plasty is well suited to other scar contractures, and the changed axis of the final scar often provides a more desirable aesthetic result in facial scar revision.

When laying out the Z-plasty, one should plot the final position of the central limb first. This final position is perpendicular to the original central limb incision and should be oriented parallel to the skin lines. Consecutive Z-plasties result in further transposition of skin and obliteration of straight-line scars. Multiple Z-plasties produce transverse shortening and lateral tension on the wound.

W-plasty

The W-plasty is similar to a Z-plasty in its ability to break up a linear scar. A defect is created by removing a scar or lesion in a precise, premarked zigzag pattern that creates multiple small triangular flaps. The multiple triangular flaps are interposed among one another. The base of each triangle is aligned with the vertex of the one opposite. Unlike the Z-plasty, the W-plasty does not confer any gain in length on

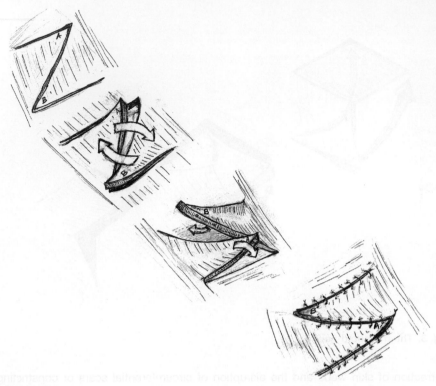

Fig. 4. Z-plasty.

the contracted scar line. As the ends of the scar are approached, the triangles should decrease in size, and the limbs of the triangles should decrease as well.

ROTATION FLAPS

Rotation flaps (**Fig. 5**)[4,13,26] are semicircular flaps raised in a subdermal plane and rotated from the donor bed around a pivot point adjacent to the defect. The defect site is visualized as a triangle with its base as the shortest side. After the flap is rotated into the defect, the donor site is closed primarily, yielding an arcuate scar. Considerable tension may be present in this flap and needs to be recognized. The line of maximal tension is directly opposite the pivot point and adjacent to the defect. Excessive tension along this line may result in ischemia and subsequent necrosis of the flap. Rotation flaps require considerable planning, and little gain is realized relative to the

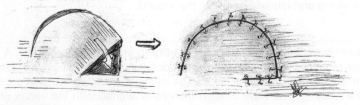

Fig. 5. Rotation flap.

size of the flap. In some cases, the donor site cannot be closed primarily and may require a skin graft. However, depending on the location of the defect, rotation flaps may be preferable to transposition or advancement flaps.

A problem with rotational flaps is the unequal length between the edge of the flap and the entire edge of the primary and secondary defects. To correct this mismatch in length, one can use the Burow's triangle technique, a cutback incision, advancement of the flap while rotating it, or suture on the bias to stretch the flap forward. The rule of thumb is that the length of the flap should be four times the width of the base of the defect. In addition, the ideal defect for repair has a height to width ratio of two to one. The blood supply is usually random, but if the surgeon designs the position of the base of the flap, it can be axial.

ADVANCEMENT FLAPS

Advancement flaps involve raising a skin paddle in a subdermal plane and moving its leading edge into the defect. The movement of the flap is longitudinal rather than rotational and is directly over the defect. Complete undermining of the flap is very important. Burow's triangles are often excised at the base of the flap to remove dog ears as the flap advances relative to the surrounding skin. These flaps have limited coverage potential and utility. The single-pedicle advancement flap is the basic flap. The ratio of defect length to flap length is one to three. Bilateral advancement flaps may be used if a single flap does not provide adequate tension-free closure of the defect.[4,13,14]

V-Y Plasty

V-Y plasty (**Fig. 6**)[27,28] is a variation of the advancement flap. In a V-Y plasty, the skin flap is not elevated and remains attached to the underlying subcutaneous tissues. A V-shaped flap is designed adjacent to the defect. The surrounding skin is elevated, and the V-shaped tissue is advanced into the wound. The donor site is closed primarily, yielding a Y-shaped closure. It may be necessary to trim the triangular edges of the leading flap to fit into the defect. This technique is particularly well suited to elongating the nasal columella and correcting the whistle deformity of the lip. The V-Y flap is one of the most versatile skin flaps and is widely used in all areas of the face.

Island Flap

Island flaps, as their name implies, involve the transposition of an island of skin that is raised on its blood supply. The skin island is moved into the defect, and the donor site is closed primarily. Often, this involves tunneling the flap under adjacent skin on its vascular pedicle. The flap island should be approximately the size of the defect to

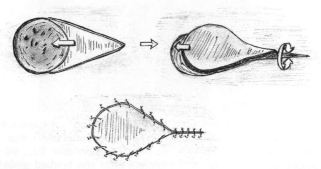

Fig. 6. V-Y advancement flap.

be covered. In areas such as the eyebrow, the island flap provides a supply of like tissue without permitting the distortion of normal anatomy. A circular island flap may pin-cushion. This complication can be avoided with proper planning.[4,13,14]

T-plasty

T-plasty is an advancement technique that converts a triangular or circular defect into an inverted-T scar. It is essentially a bilateral advancement flap and works well in the central forehead, above the eyebrows, and on the upper lip just above the vermilion. Care must be taken, because the vertical limb of the T can be noticeable in some areas.[13]

CLINICAL SCENARIOS

Many options are available for closing defects of the face and other areas of the body; the authors outline only a few of them here. The reconstruction of each defect must be individualized to attain the optimal aesthetic outcome. In each of the following clinical cases, multiple skin flap options are discussed for each defect. These are, of course, not the only options, and the selected reconstruction is not the only good choice. The principles of selecting an appropriate repair are the same in each case.

Fig. 7A depicts a 65-year-old woman who underwent excision of basal cell carcinoma and now has a 2.5-cm defect in the side of her nose. Aesthetic reconstruction of nasal deficits is a common problem posed to the reconstructive surgeon by the high

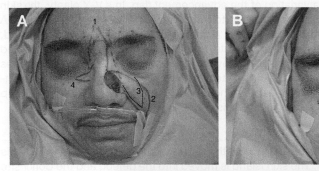

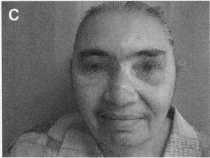

Fig. 7. (*A*) A 65-year-old woman who underwent excision of basal cell carcinoma with a 2.5-cm defect in the side of the nose. (1) Transposition glabelar flap. (2) Advancement flap following the nasolabial groove medially. (3) Nasolabial flap. (4) Bilobed glabelar flap. (*B*) Intraoperative photograph of patient after the bilobed glabelar flap with the donor site closed in a Y-fashion. (*C*) Postoperative photograph of the bilobed glabelar flap.

incidence of nasal skin cancer. Several considerations need to be addressed in the reconstruction of nasal defects: color and texture match, minimization of bulkiness, appreciation of discrete aesthetic units of the nose, skin tension lines and wrinkles, adequacy of tissue, and vascularity.

The glabelar skin offers an excellent source of tissue for nasal repairs. The transposition glabelar flap provides good skin match and adequate skin to cover this defect, and the glabelar region can be closed primarily with a vertical scar orientation at the donor site that can be easily camouflaged.

The incision can be made along the nasolabial groove and along the cheek, following natural skin lines, to raise an advancement flap. This flap is advanced medially to cover the defect. The cheek has good skin laxity to close the defect at its base. However, the bulkiness of the cheek relative to the nasal skin may be obvious.

A nasolabial flap[29] can be elevated in the subcutaneous plane of the cheek and transposed to the defect. In this case, a dog ear needs to be excised at the pivot point superiorly. The cheek has to be undermined beyond the flap to allow for transposition of this flap. The donor site can be closed primarily, with the closure falling along the nasolabial fold. Closure of the donor site would disrupt the eyelid-cheek skin lines.

A bilobed glabelar flap can be used, as in this case (**Fig. 7**B), to cover the defect. The smaller lobe is transposed to cover the donor defect. The rest of the glabelar region site can be closed primarily in a Y fashion. Good skin color and texture match are seen, with minimal tension and good camouflage of scars (**Fig. 7**C).

Fig. 8A shows a 62-year-old man with a cheek defect after resection of squamous cell carcinoma. The defect is 4.5 cm in size and lies 3.5 cm lateral to the mouth.

An advancement flap may be designed, based either laterally or inferiorly, to close this defect. Parallel incisions can be made, raised in the subcutaneous plane, and advanced to cover the defect. Good laxity of the skin of the cheek, especially in the elderly, provides sufficient tissue for the repair. Dog ears at the base of the flap can be excised. The inferiorly based advancement flap takes advantage of the laxity of the skin of the neck, and the scar lines fall in the natural skin lines. Hence, the inferiorly based advancement flap is a better option than the laterally based one.

A banner flap can also be used to transpose into the defect. However, the scar may not be as easily camouflaged.

Other options include (1) a cheek rotation flap, (2) a rhomboid flap inferiorly based to take advantage of the lax skin of the neck, and (3) a V-Y advancement flap based laterally (**Figs. 8**B and **8C**).[30,31]

In the patient shown in **Fig. 9**A, the defect is centrally located in the dorsum of the nose. Several good options are available for its reconstruction.

A superiorly based V-Y advancement flap may be used.

A rotation glabelar flap may be used and a backcut designed to close the donor site pivot point in a Y configuration (**Fig. 9**B).[32]

A rhomboid flap would not be the ideal design, because the nasal skin is not as mobile and may distort the medial canthus and create a web or ectropion. It is important that the design of the flap in this patient lie within the wrinkles of the face to mask the scar and not distort the eyebrows and eyes.

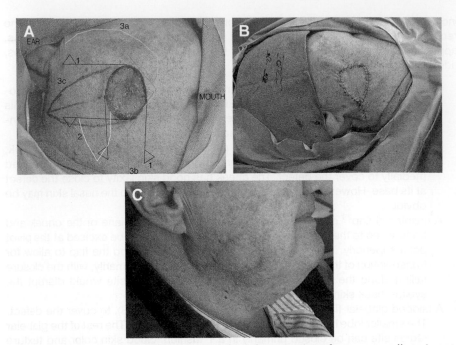

Fig. 8. (A) A 62-year-old man with a cheek defect after resection of squamous cell carcinoma 4.5 cm in size. (1) Advancement flap based laterally or inferiorly with excision of Burow's triangles. (2) Banner flap. (3a) Cheek rotation flap. (3b) Rhomboid flap. (3c) V-Y advancement flap. (B) Intraoperative photograph of patient after the V-Y advancement flap of the cheek defect. (C) Postoperative photograph of patient after the V-Y advancement flap of the cheek defect.

A banner flap may also be designed, using the tissue available from the side wall of the nose and primary closure of the donor site.

Fig. 10A shows an 85-year-old woman after resection of basal cell carcinoma from her upper lip, creating a 1.5-cm circular defect. This defect lies just above the vermilion and medial to the nasolabial fold and is close to the alar base, philtrum, and cupid's bow.

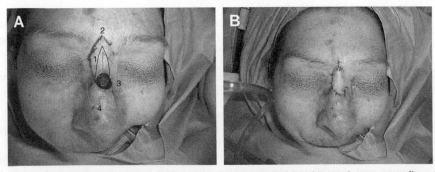

Fig. 9. (A) Patient with a dorsal nose defect. (1) Superiorly based V-Y advancement flap. (2) Rotation glabelar flap and a backcut to close the donor site. (3) Rhomboid flap. (4) Banner flap. (B) Intraoperative photograph of rotation glabelar flap with a backcut to close the donor site in a Y-fashion.

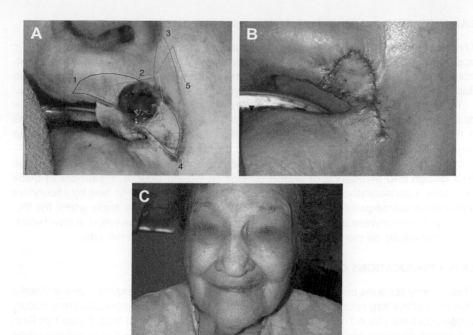

Fig. 10. (*A*) An 85-year-old female after resection of basal cell carcinoma from the upper lip with a 1.5-cm defect resulting. (1) Bilateral V-Y advancement flap. (2) A-T advancement flap. (3) Nasolabial flap. (4) Single V-Y advancement along the nasolabial fold and vermilion border. (5) Rhomboid flap would distort the nasolabial fold to a greater degree than the other flaps mentioned. (*B*) Intraoperative photograph of V-Y advancement flap in the upper lip. (*C*) Postoperative photograph of V-Y advancement flap.

A bilateral V-Y advancement flap may be used to close the defect with adequate undermining. Excellent laxity of the skin and natural skin folds and wrinkles are present and may be used to the surgeon's advantage. However, the medial V-Y flap may distort the cupid's bow.

An A-T advancement flap may also be used, by taking a triangular wedge out superiorly from the defect and undermining on both sides to close the defect.

A nasolabial flap may be used by raising the flap along the nasolabial fold.

A single V-Y advancement flap was designed, following the vermilion border and the nasolabial fold to advance medially into the defect (**Figs. 10**B and **10**C).[33]

A rhomboid flap, in this case, would distort the nasolabial fold and would not mask the scar as well.

FOLLOW-UP CARE

Follow-up care is an important aspect of the treatment of any surgical wound. Suture removal is timed to prevent suture cross marks and epithelial cysts. Patients need to be advised as to the proper management of new scars and monitored to ensure that the healing process is progressing normally. As in the treatment of any condition, follow-up and continuity of care are vital aspects of good medical practice. Skin flaps take 3 to 6 months to mature. They tend to look puffy and distorted at first but will settle down and improve over time. Patients need to be reassured.

EARLY COMPLICATIONS OF FLAP RECONSTRUCTION

The possible complications after flap reconstruction vary in severity and require distinct approaches depending on their type. Fortunately, most of the complications are preventable as well as amenable to treatment. The most common early complications after skin flap reconstruction surgery are infection, hematoma, seroma, and wound dehiscence.

The complication of flap necrosis is more serious and is usually due to a design flaw or an error in execution of the reconstruction. These errors include the use of too small a flap for a given defect, damage to the flap's blood supply, extension of the flap beyond its blood supply, or closure of the defect in such a way that it is subject to too much tension. Flap necrosis may usually be avoided by means of more precise flap design and avoidance of undue tension on wound closure. Treatment of distal necrosis is conservative and may include allowing certain areas to heal by secondary intention or subsequent surgical revision of the area. However, in areas where the flap was placed to prevent a deforming scar contracture, such as the eyelid, a new reconstruction should be performed as soon as the wound condition permits.

LATE COMPLICATIONS OF FLAP RECONSTRUCTION

These complications are avoided for the most part by means of experience and careful planning of the flap reconstruction. Unfavorable scarring is a complication that occurs when scars are placed outside of the direction of the skin tension lines. Scars that lie in the wrong direction may be revised with a Z-plasty or a W-plasty. Pin-cushioning (trap door deformity) of the flap is another complication that arises from a curvilinear scar. Correction of the pin-cushion deformity should not be performed until the scar matures. Options for correction include excision of the old scar, defatting of the flap, and closure with Z-plasties or a W-plasty.

Hypertrophic scars are uncommon on the face. However, keloids can be a major concern. Any patient with a personal or family history of keloids or a personal history of hypertrophic scars must be warned about the risk of developing additional keloids or hypertrophic scars. Once a keloid forms, many treatment options are available, most of which are only partially effective in minimizing the scar. Pressure, topical silicone, steroid injections, and massage are the standard treatments, although re-excision in conjunction with intralesional steroids and postoperative radiation may also be considered for unresponsive lesions.

OUTCOME AND PROGNOSIS

When local flaps are insufficient to cover a wound properly, distant tissue may be imported using techniques such as skin grafting, pedicled flaps, axial flaps, fasciocutaneous flaps, myocutaneous flaps, and free flaps. If the removal of sutures that are too tight or the correction of a hematoma delays the repair, this is a small price to pay for the avoidance of flap necrosis and a better end-result. The primary goal in tumor surgery is adequate treatment of the tumor. Only after that treatment may a definitive reconstruction be undertaken. The reconstruction must preserve function and provide the best possible cosmetic result.

ACKNOWLEDGMENTS

Special thanks to Dr Gordon Kaplan, Plastic Surgery Resident, UMDNJ/New Jersey Medical School, for his artistic contribution to this manuscript and to Michelle Granick for providing her expertise with the digital photographs.

REFERENCES

1. Converse JM. Introduction to plastic surgery. In: Converse JM, editor. 2nd edition. Reconstructive plastic surgery, Vol. 1. Philadelphia: WB Saunders; 1977. p. 3–68.
2. McGregor IA. Design of skin flaps. Lancet 1970;2(2):130–3.
3. McGregor IA, Morgan G. Axial and random pattern flaps. Br J Plast Surg 1973;26: 202–13.
4. Place MJ, Herber SC, Hardesty RA. Basic techniques and principles in plastic surgery. In: Grabb and Smith's Plastic Surgery. 5th edition. Boston: Lippincott-Raven; 1997. p. 13–26.
5. Lamberty BGH, Healy C. Flaps: physiology, principles of design, and pitfalls. In: Cohen M, editor, Mastery of plastic and reconstructive surgery, Vol. 1. Boston: Little, Brown and Co.; 1994. p. 56–70.
6. Daniel RK, Williams HB. The free transfer of skin flaps by microvascular anastomoses: an experimental study and a reappraisal. Part I: the vascular supply of the skin. Plast Reconstr Surg 1973;52:16–31.
7. Webster JP. Thoraco-epigastric tubed pedicles. Surg Clin North Am 1937;17:145.
8. Kunert P. Structure and construction: the system of skin flaps. Ann Plast Surg 1991;27:509–16.
9. Cormack GC, Lamberty BGH. A classification of fasciocutaneous flaps according to their patterns of vascularization. Br J Plast Surg 1984;37:80–7.
10. Daniel RK, Kerrigan CL. Principles and physiology of skin flaps. In: McCarthy JG, editor, Plastic surgery, Vol. 1. Philadelphia: WB Saunders; 1990. p. 275–328.
11. Kayser MR, Hodges PL. Surgical flaps. In: Barton FE Jr, editor. Selected readings in plastic surgery. Vol. 8, No. 3. Dallas (TX): Baylor University Medical Center; 1995. p. 1–58.
12. Taylor GI. The blood supply of the skin. In: Grabb and Smith's Plastic Surgery. 5th edition. Boston: Lippincott-Raven; 1997. p. 47–60.
13. Baker SR, Swanson NA. Local flaps in facial reconstruction. St. Louis: Mosby; 1995.
14. Jackson IT. Local flaps in head and neck reconstruction. St. Louis: Quality Medical Publishing; 1985.
15. Masson JK, Mendelson BC. The banner flap. Am J Surg 1977;134(3):419–23.
16. Zitelli JA. The bilobed flap for nasal reconstruction. Arch Dermatol 1989;125(7): 957–9.
17. McGregor JC, Soutar DS. A critical assessment of the bilobed flap. Br J Plast Surg 1981;34(2):197–205.
18. Golcman R, Speranzini MB, Golcman B. The bilobed island flap in nasal ala reconstruction. Br J Plast Surg 1998;51(7):493–8.
19. Zimany A. The bi-lobed flap. Facial Plast Surg Clin North Am 1953;11:424–34.
20. Morgan BL, Samiian MR. Advantages of the bilobed flap for closure of small defects of the face. Plast Reconstr Surg 1973;52(1):35–7.
21. Bray DA. Clinical applications of the rhomboid flap. Arch Otolaryngol 1983; 109(1):37–42.
22. Borges AF. The rhombic flap. Plast Reconstr Surg 1981;67(4):458–66.
23. Borges AF. Choosing the correct Limberg flap. Plast Reconstr Surg 1978;62(4): 542–5.
24. Becker FF. Rhomboid flap in facial reconstruction. New concept of tension lines. Arch Otolaryngol 1979;105(10):569–73.
25. Lober CW, Mendelsohn HE, Fenske NA. Rhomboid transposition flaps. Aesthetic Plast Surg 1985;9(2):121–4.

26. Green RK, Angelats J. A full nasal skin rotation flap for closure of soft-tissue defects in the lower one-third of the nose. Plast Reconstr Surg 1996;98(1):163–6.
27. Cronin TD. The V-Y rotational flap for nasal tip defects. Ann Plast Surg 1983;11(4): 282–8.
28. Omidi MS, Granick MS. The versatile V-Y flap for facial reconstruction. Dermatol Surg 2004;30(3):415–20.
29. Zitelli JA. The nasolabial flap as a single-stage procedure. Arch Dermatol 1990; 126(11):1445–8.
30. Schrudde J, Beinhoff U. Reconstruction of the face by means of the angle-rotation flap. Aesthetic Plast Surg 1987;11(1):15–22.
31. Yotsuyanagi T, Yamashita K, Urushidate S, et al. Reconstruction of large nasal defects with a combination of loca flaps based on the aesthetic subunit principle. Plast Reconstr Surg 2001;107(6):1358–62.
32. Rigg BM. The dorsal nasal flap. Plast Reconstr Surg 1973;52(4):361–4.
33. Carvalho LM, Ramos RR, Santos ID, et al. V-Y advancement flap for the reconstruction of partial and full thickness defects of the upper lip. Scand J Plast Reconstr Surg Hand Surg 2002;36(1):28–33.

The Culture of Safety

Deborah S. Hickman Mathis, RN, MS, CNOR, RNFA

KEYWORDS

• Safety • Error reduction • Nursing standards

SAFETY

It is the cornerstone of perioperative nursing. It is the responsibility of the perioperative team to continuously monitor the quality of care provided to each patient. AORN states, "A fundamental precept of AORN is that it is the responsibility of professional Registered Nurses to ensure safe, high- quality nursing care to patients undergoing operative and other invasive procedures."

Safety is not a new effort for healthcare providers, but for many consumers of healthcare normal apprehension has escalated to fear. Their concern had substance with the publishing of "To Err Is Human, Building a Safer Health System," in 2000, by Linda T. Kohn, Janet M. Corrigan, and Molla S. Donaldson. This one article was a catalyst to position healthcare under new analysis.

On June 14, 2006, The Institute for Healthcare Improvement and its partner organizations came together to launch the 100,000 Lives Campaign, a national effort to reduce preventable deaths in U.S. hospitals. No one could have imagined the strength of the response. An extraordinary resurgence of spirit and an unprecedented commitment to change and collaboration across the health care industry evolved. A renewed national commitment to improve patient safety through this initiative was so successful that the IHI set a new goal "Protect patients from five million incidents of medical harm over the next two years (December 2006–December 2008)." The 5 Million Lives Campaign challenged American hospitals to adopt 12 changes in care that save lives and reduce patient injuries.

Each year the Joint Commission has expanded on the 12 changes suggested by the IHI. The National Patient Safety Goals program provides a significant focus on patient safety within health care. Adherence to the program is mandatory for more than 15,000 Joint Commission-accredited healthcare organizations. It is designed to stimulate healthcare organizational improvement activities for several of the most pressing patient safety issues that all organizations are struggling to manage effectively.

Oversight of the National Patient Safety Goals is rigorous and the ongoing evolution of this program is a reflection of how complex the processes of health care are to change before sustainable improvements in patient safety can occur.

Healthcare providers at all levels are required to quantify (scientific assessment), evaluate the data (plan), (implement) changes with measurable criteria to (evaluate),

Renue Plastic Surgery, Renue Surgery Center, 2500 Starling Street, Suite 604, Brunswick, GA 31520, USA
E-mail address: debbie@renuemd.com

Perioperative Nursing Clinics 6 (2011) 187–193
doi:10.1016/j.cpen.2011.04.003
1556-7931/11/$ – see front matter © 2011 Elsevier Inc. All rights reserved.

with additional elements of oversight (CMS, JCAHO, AAAHC, State, WHO, etc.). This is the core of healthcare provision and nursing practice.

It is for these reasons that all healthcare providers must be able to clearly communicate this to their patients, families, employers, payers, and regulatory agencies.

HOW DO YOU BEGIN?

First, healthcare providers must be knowledgeable and able to articulate what they as practitioners do each day to keep their patients safe. They must understand the relevance of their individual practice to the whole. They must be educated as to the above and understand their role.

My academic nursing curriculum covered Perioperative Nursing from the perspective of an experience, with a focusing on in-patient hospital pre and post-operative patient care. Working as a Surgical Technician during nursing school my goal was to be a perioperative nurse, but I felt pressure from professors, peers, and even the human resource department to be a "real nurse" first. "Start on the floor first, then work your way to the ICUs," they would advise. It was at that point the "passion" to teach others what Perioperative Nurses contribute to the Perioperative Team was fueled. I wanted to help nurses articulate what "nursing" means to the patient undergoing surgery. We are patient advocates.

Fast forward, years of experience, higher education and holding leadership positions, has never diminished that early passion for the core nursing role as the patient safety advocate. As a current healthcare leader it is my responsibility to educate the entire perioperative team about this enormous topic of SAFETY. Privately, I asked, "How do you do that?"

The answer was conceived while I was the Director of Surgical Services at our local hospital, and implemented while serving as the Director of Surgical Services for Renue Plastic Surgery, a free-standing plastic/cosmetic and reconstructive ambulatory surgery center. The concept was to simply break down the care we render every day utilizing the National Patient Safety Goals.

We named our program "Surgical Services; A Culture of Safety."

The program was simple but inclusive to patient safety in the perioperative setting:

1. Draft a policy with the intention to communicate "The Culture of Safety" in an atmosphere where all members of the Perioperative Team can openly express concerns, report errors, and discuss process improvements without fear of reprisal.
2. Define and publish the procedures/tools that the organization has in place to ensure safety. These can be
   a. "Hand-Off Communication" Tools to communicate important patient information between team members
   b. Pre-Procedural "Check-Lists" to verify the correct patient, procedure, surgical site, all necessary test(s) completed and results communicated, equipment and supplies immediately available, etc.
   c. Scripted "Time-Out" verification that is interactive, multidisciplinary, and consistent in elements
   d. "Concern Reports" to allow staff to communicate in writing any issue that distracts or hinders safe patient care
   e. "Concern Response Form" vital to communicate back to the staff member resolution or course of action taken regarding their written concern report.
   f. "Risk Management Variance Reports" for those events of defined serious nature.
   g. "Educational Calendar" published after input from staff and other team members to meet the annual education needs of the staff to include competencies, high risk or low volume problem prone areas, new equipment, etc.

h. "Monthly Staff Meetings" A monthly meeting between Renue Surgery Center and Renue Plastic Surgery team members is conducted to meet the educational needs of the staff including competencies, drills, new equipment, regulations, pertinent journal articles, etc.

i. "Quarterly Governing Board Meetings" to share our programs with all stakeholders

3. Address each National Patient Safety Goal with the intent to promote specific improvements in patient safety. Express this to each practitioner and staff member by clearly indentifying their individual roles and practice expectations among the perioperative team.

a. Improve the Accuracy of Patient Identification:
   i. Perioperative Implication- Identify the patient prior to any procedure of surgery using their name and date of birth.

b. Improve the Effectiveness of Communication among Caregivers:
   i. Perioperative Implication- Verbal patient handoff in the transition of patient care. Also, staff members will read back and verify any verbal orders or critical lab values. Written communication will only use an approved list of abbreviations.

c. Improve the Safety of Obtaining and giving Medications:
   i. Perioperative Implications: Label all medications and solutions on and off the sterile field. Keep the original container until the end of the procedure. Verbally and visually verify medications. Any medications or solutions found unlabeled are discarded immediately.

d. Reduce the Risk of Health Care Associated Infections:
   i. Perioperative Implication- Reconcile medications when patients are admitted and discharged from the facility. If a patient is transferred, and updated medication reconciliation list is included with the verbal hand off information.

e. Reduce the Risk of Patient Harm Resulting from Falls:
   i. Perioperative Implication- Any patient in the surgical suite is considered at a high risk for falls. In addition to Standard Fall Precautions, every health care provider will:
      1. Maintain a low caregiver to patient ratio
      2. Position patient within the line of sight of team members
      3. Assist patient in and out of the stretcher and remain with the patient when assisted to the restroom.
      4. Frequent patient checks by team members.

f. Encourage the Patient's Active Involvement in their own Care as a Safety Strategy:
   i. Perioperative Implication- Encourage active participation of the patent and patient's family in the site marking process, encourage patients to "speak up" with their concerns about personal care.
      1. Renue Surgery Center identifies safety risks inherent in its patient population

g. Improve Recognition and Response to Changes in a Patient's Condition:
   i. Perioperative Implication- Monitor physiological changes: report blood loss, changes in vital signs, equipment functionality, etc.

h. The Organization Meets the Expectations of the Universal Protocol:
   i. Perioperative Implication- Preoperative verification of the correct patient, procedure and procedure site is done by the preoperative RN. The official time out is performed immediately prior to incision.
      1. Acute MI
      2. Heart Failure
      3. Pneumonia
      4. Surgical Care Improvement Project- SCIP.

    i. Prophylactic antibiotic received prior to surgical incision:
       i. Perioperative Implication- Anesthesia personnel ensure that the antibiotic is available and given prior to incision and documents it in the Anesthesia Record.
    j. Proper prophylactic antibiotic selection for surgical patients:
       i. Perioperative Implication- Preoperative nurses and Anesthesia personnel verify that the patient has no allergies to the recommended medications.
    k. Prophylactic antibiotics discontinued within 24 hours after surgery:
       i. Perioperative Implication- PACU nurses verify the antibiotic was given in the OR. If the patient is transferred to an acute care facility, nurses verify that the antibiotic orders do not exceed 24 hours unless an active infection is documented.
    l. Cardiac patients have controlled 6 a.m. postoperative serum glucose levels.
    m. Appropriate hair removal with surgery patients:
       i. Perioperative Implication- OR nurses must document hair removal (NO shaving)
    n. Immediate postoperative Normothermia:
       i. Perioperative Implication- Preoperatively, nurses use Bair Paws for patients or if hypothermic on arrival, OR nurses ensure proper use of Bair Hugger blankets and warmed blankets. PACU nurses use Bair Paws on patients that are hypothermic.
    o. Surgery patients with recommended venous thromboembolism prophylaxis ordered:
       i. Perioperative Implication- SCDs placed to bilateral legs in the OR.
4. Mentor, Lecture, Provide Written Material, Post Information, Live It, Model It!
    a. Back to the basics- AORN Standards- Recommended Practices and Guidelines:
    b. Surgical Attire and PPE
       i. Freshly laundered scrubs from home must be brought in a plastic bag and changed into at Renue Surgery Center. Scrubs changed daily.
       ii. Cover all head and facial hair. Washable cloth scrub hats are covered by a disposable cap.
       iii. Wear masks in the presence of open sterile supplies, cover the mouth and nose to prevent venting, change all surgical attire after each case.
       iv. Confine all jewelry in the scrub attire, if scrubbing a case, all rings, watches and bracelets are removed, and earrings are confined in the scrub hat or removed.
       v. Fingernails are kept short, clean, natural and healthy. Use a nail cleaner under running water prior to the first case each day.
       vi. Protective eyewear, mask or face shield must be worn when splashing or spraying can occur (always).
       vii. Gowns and gloves are PPE and should be worn when spills and fluids are likely. Both must be removed before leaving the OR.
       viii. Any ancillary staff members, who must enter the semi-restricted areas, are required to use a clean jumpsuit over their clothes or change into surgical approved scrubs. Approval given by OR Director.
       ix. Vendors will wear clean, freshly laundered scrubs. No personal outside scrubs will be allowed in the OR suite.
    c. Infection Control
       i. *Hand Hygiene-* the single most important step in the prevention of infections- All personnel should practice general hand hygiene before and after patient contact, after removing gloves, and any time there is a possibility that there has been contact with blood or infected material.
       ii. VISIBLE SOIL- wash with soap and water

   iii. NO VISIBLE SOIL- sanitize with alcohol-based rub or soap and water

   iv. Surgical Hand Antisepsis- the antiseptic surgical scrub or antiseptic hand rub is to be performed or applied before donning sterile attire.

   v. Surgical Scrub

   vi. Wash hands, wash forearms and clean nails with a disposable nail cleaner before beginning the scrub.

  vii. Visualize each finger, bilateral hands and arms as having four sides. Scrub all four sides effectively using a count or timed approved method.

 viii. Hands are held higher than elbows during the scrub. Hands and arms are to be dried with a sterile towel.

   ix. Surgical Hand Rub- the antiseptic surgical scrub or antiseptic hand rub is to be performed or applied before donning sterile attire.

   x. Wash hands, wash forearms and clean nails with a disposable nail cleaner before beginning the scrub.

   xi. Dry hands.

  xii. Dispense the recommended amount of product, apply hand rub to hands and forearms and let the product dry thoroughly before donning sterile gown and gloves.

 xiii. Standard Precautions- should be used when caring for all patients in the perioperative setting.

 xiv. *Healthcare Workers*:
   1. Must receive Hep B immunizations unless medically contraindicated
   2. Work practices should minimize risk of exposure to infection.
   3. Workers with weeping lesions or dermatitis should refrain from providing direct patient care.

  xv. *Traffic Patterns*:

 xvi. OR is secure and ID badges worn by anyone entering Renue Surgery Center

 xvii. Movement of personnel should be kept to a minimum to reduce airborne contamination while procedures are in progress.

xviii. Doors to the OR should remain closed to maintain proper air flow, temperature and pressure.

 xix. *Maintaining the sterile field*

  xx. Scrubbed personnel should don sterile attire away from the sterile field to prevent contamination

 xxi. The front of the gown is sterile to the level of the sterile field

 xxii. Gown sleeves are sterile from two inches above the elbow to the cuff

xxiii. The neckline, shoulders, armpits and gown backs are considered non-sterile and once hands pass beyond the cuff then the cuff is considered contaminated.

xxiv. Ensure that only sterile items are delivered to the sterile field by inspecting packaging, expiration dates, processing seal and sterilization indicator.

 xxv. Rigid container systems should be opened on a separate surface with the lid lifted toward the person opening the container . Also the filter needs to be checked.

xxvi. The contents of the rigid container are removed and placed on the sterile field after the scrubbed person has donned sterile attire.

xxvii. All items introduced to the sterile field should be opened, dispensed and transferred by methods that maintain sterility

xxviii. Un-scrubbed personnel should open wrapped sterile supplies by opening the wrapper flap furthest away from the body first, followed by the right and left sides, and the nearest flap will be opened last with all edges secured.

xxix. Sterile items should be presented to the scrubbed person or placed securely on the sterile field.

xxx. Sharp and heavy objects should be presented to the scrubbed person or opened on a separate surface.

xxxi. Peel pouches should be presented to the scrubbed person to prevent contamination of the package contents.

xxxii. Solutions are dispensed into a labeled receptacle on the sterile field near the edge of the table, or held by the scrubbed person, and poured slowly to avoid splashing. Any remaining fluid is considered contaminated and should be discarded.

xxxiii. Medications are delivered to the sterile field without removing the stoppers for the purpose of pouring. A sterile transfer device should be used.

xxxiv. An open sterile field requires continuous visual observation and should be prepared as close as possible to the time of use. Sterile fields are never covered and/or left unattended.

xxxv. All personnel moving in and around the sterile field should do so in a manner that maintains the sterile field.

xxxvi. Scrubbed personnel should remain close to the sterile field.

xxxvii. Scrubbed personnel should not leave the OR for flashed supplies

xxxviii. Un-scrubbed personnel should face the sterile field and not walk between two sterile fields

xxxix. When a break in technique occurs, corrective action should be taken immediately. If the break cannot be corrected, it should be reported and recorded.

xl. *Sterilization*

xli. Instrument Reprocessing

xlii. You can clean without sterilization but you can NEVER sterilize without cleaning.

xliii. Effective sterilization cannot take place without effective cleaning.

xliv. Do not take shortcuts in the cleaning process of instrumentation needing to be reprocessed between cases due to pressure for a rapid room turnover.

xlv. (Loaner Instruments and Trays)

xlvi. NEVER bring a processed tray processed outside of the facility directly to your sterile field

xlvii. All loaner instruments are considered contaminated and should be delivered directly to decontamination for processing.

xlviii. Flash sterilization should not be used as a substitute for late delivery of loaner instrumentation.

xlix. *Environmental Responsibilities*

l. Conscientious adherence to cleaning and disinfecting procedures is crucial for the prevention and transmission of infection.

li. (Preoperative Procedures)

lii. The patient should be provided a clean, safe environment

liii. All horizontal surfaces in the OR/procedural areas should be dusted with a damp cloth before the first scheduled procedure of the day. This is to include furniture, surgical lights, equipment, etc.

liv. (Intraoperative Procedures)

lv. Preparation of the OR/ procedural area includes a visual inspection for cleanliness before the case cart or any supplies are brought into the room

lvi. Clean spills or splatters as they occur with a disinfected wipe (no sprays during a procedure)

lvii. Contain contaminated discarded sponges in a manner that facilitates visualization during counting.

lviii. Closing of OR following contaminated or dirty procedures (Class III or IV) is not necessary when cleaned properly unless suspected of CJD (Mad cow disease)

lix. (Postoperative Procedures)

lx. A clean safe environment should be re-established after each procedure.

lxi. Place trash and laundry in the appropriate containers (red bags vs. clear bags)

lxii. Clean all horizontal surfaces and receptacles, clean all nonporous surfaces such as mattresses and pillows, safety straps, arm boards, etc. on both sides.

lxiii. Mop under OR bed and in a 3 foot parameter and further if contamination has occurred

lxiv. Change mop heads after each use

lxv. (Anesthesia Equipment)

lxvi. Single use items are discarded after use.

lxvii. Reusable equipment that comes in contact with mucous membranes (Laryngoscope blades, etc.) should be cleaned and reprocessed by high level disinfection (Steris) or sterilization (Flash)

lxviii. Equipment that comes in contact with intact skin (EKG leads, Pulse Oximeter probe, BP cuff etc.) should be cleaned between use on patients with an approved disinfectant

lxix. Surfaces of anesthesia equipment (machines and knobs) touched by personnel while providing patient care should be cleaned between patient uses with an approved disinfectant.

Index

Note: Page numbers of article titles are in **boldface** type.

Perioperative Nursing Clinics 6 (2011) 195–200
doi:10.1016/S1556-7931(11)00018-0
1556-7931/11/$ – see front matter © 2011 Elsevier Inc. All rights reserved.

periopnursing.theclinics.com